Writing:
A Guide for Therapists

Skills for Practice Series

Series editors: Sally French and Jo Laing

Titles published

In preparation

• Skills for Practice •

Writing:
A Guide for Therapists
by

Sally French

BSc, MSc(psych), MSc(soc), GradDipPhys, DipTP
Lecturer, School of Health, Welfare and Community
Education, Open University, UK

and

Julius Sim

BA, MSc, MCSP
Principal Lecturer, School of Health and Social Sciences,
Coventry University, UK

BUTTERWORTH
HEINEMANN

Butterworth-Heinemann Ltd
Linacre House, Jordan Hill, Oxford OX2 8DP

℞ A member of the Reed Elsevier group

OXFORD   LONDON   BOSTON
MUNICH   NEW DELHI   SINGAPORE   SYDNEY
TOKYO   TORONTO   WELLINGTON

First published 1993

British Library Cataloguing in Publication Data
French, Sally
  Writing: Guide for Therapists. – (Skills
  for Practice Series)
  I. Title   II. Sim, Julius   III. Series
  808.0666158

ISBN 0-7506 0580 4

Library of Congress Cataloguing in Publication Data
French, Sally.
    Writing: a guide for therapists/by Sally French and Julius Sim.
      p.   cm.—(Skills for practice series)
    Includes bibliographical references and index.
    ISBN 0–7506–0580–4
    1. Psychotherapy—Authorship.   I. Sim, Julius.   II. Title.
III. Series.
RC437.2.F733   1993
808'.066616—dc20   93–24425
                                                              CIP

Printed and bound in Great Britain by Biddles Ltd Guildford and
Kings Lynn

Contents

Preface

Over the years, therapists and therapy students have become involved in a larger range of writing tasks in both their course work and their clinical practice. They are expected to write clinical reports, patient instructions, research reports, student assessments, papers for publication and essays and examinations. These activities require therapists to write in varied styles with different readers in mind – patients, examiners and colleagues from their own and other professions.

Writing is a skill and, like all skills, can be improved upon with knowledge and practice. The aim of this book is to provide therapists and therapy students with the necessary information and guidance to help them succeed in all aspects of their writing. The book has a practical orientation discussing, for example the writing of research reports, essays, clinical notes and papers for publication. The use of bibliographic references, the publishing process and the use of graphics are also discussed, as well as the issues of style, the writing process and stereotypical language. Every effort has been made to ensure that the contents of the book are accessible. It is extensively referenced to assist those readers who require further information.

We would like to thank all our friends and colleagues who have helped and encouraged us to write this book. Particular thanks are extended to Jackie Waterfield of the School of Health and Social Sciences, Coventry University, to Christine Wright of the School of Mathematical and Information Sciences, Coventry University and to Caroline Makepeace of Butterworth-Heinemann for her constant encouragement and good humour. Nicholas Reville LLB, MA, Solr, Senior Lecturer in Law, De Monfort University, provided much help and advice concerning chapter 10, for which the authors are most grateful. Thanks are also extended to Lawrence Erlbaum Associates for their permission to adapt chapter 6 from the following publication: Sim J. (1989) The use of bibliographic references. *Physiotherapy Practice* 5, 25–32. The authors take full responsibility for any errors or omissions in the text.

We hope that this book will encourage therapists to communicate their thoughts, knowledge and ideas in writing, for the benefit of patients and clients, their colleagues and the therapy professions as a whole.

Sally French
Julius Sim

1

Writing to Communicate

When any of us read a text, we have, if that text is well written, received a communication from the person who wrote it. If the writer has made the content clear then its purpose, that of communicating certain ideas or information, will be achieved. We all know how pleasing it is to find that a passage is easily read and informative, especially if it is elegantly written. We also know the frustration of trying to tease the meaning from a passage that is full of jargon, badly translated or ambiguous.

Writing, unlike the spoken word, is 'permanent, spatial and visual' (Garton and Pratt, 1989: 4) and has long had a political significance because it may contain and convey powerful ideas. We have all heard that 'the pen is mightier than the sword'. There is liberty in self expression and the exchange of ideas; we need only to think how hard the privileged classes of many societies have fought over the centuries to make sure that underprivileged people remained illiterate, to realize that we are dealing with a powerful medium. We have, more recently, become aware of how we can oppress others with writing. Few of us wish to be seen publicly as racist or sexist, for example, yet our writing can sometimes display bigotry that we hardly knew we possessed (see chapter 3).

Even in our everyday lives, writing often has more significance than the spoken word. The latter is ephemeral and transient. We can change it, we can say 'No, that's not what I meant', we can deny that something was said or suggest that we have been misheard or misquoted. We know that if we want absolute confirmation of anything in our everyday lives we 'get it in writing'. We need receipts for things we buy, contracts for our jobs of work, confirmation by letter of decisions reached on the telephone. Writing differs also from the spoken word in that it does not carry with it supportive body language such as facial expression or posture.

In these days, our society requires a higher degree of literacy from all of us if we are to operate successfully within it. Professional people are required increasingly to be accountable in writing for their actions. Their clients and students, now more confident and articulate than formerly, may wish, and have the right, to know what is being written about them. In addition, in an increasingly open society, the written word is becoming less and less confidential to the work environment. For all these reasons, writers may be anxious that their writing is correct and that it will not later incriminate them in some way.

Choices and assumptions

Vocabulary

When any of us starts to write, we need to make choices and assumptions. We might assume, for example, that we have a shared vocabulary but, for any two people, even those speaking the same native tongue, this will be partial. We may not, for instance, share each other's technical terms. Even terms as familiar to therapists as 'admission' and 'discharge' may cause confusion among patients. The former might refer to an entrance fee or a confession, and the latter to a bodily excretion or a dismissal. On the other hand, one therapist would not write to another of 'paralysis down one side' but would use the term 'hemiplegia'.

Style

Further choices will be made by the writer concerning the style to adopt when writing. This will depend upon the purpose that the writing has, the topic with which it is dealing, and the writer's knowledge of and relationship with the reader. Thus, the answer to an examination question will have an entirely different style from that of a letter to a friend, even if the two are written by the same person.

Some of our writing is, of course, just for ourselves. A person may write a diary that is seen by no one else but may enjoy, years later, reading it and remembering those earlier experiences. A student may take notes at a lecture which need to be easily read and understood later. Someone may make a shopping list or a list of reminders. In these instances, the writer and reader are one; the shared experience is identical at the time of writing. Because of this, the writing might be almost meaningless to anyone else, but still make perfect sense to the person who wrote it.

Within one written document, the writing may move through a variety of styles. In a letter to a friend the words might run something like this 'Saw Ellen yesterday, she sends her love. She was with her latest man – good looking, tall, bearded. They were off Christmas shopping. I didn't like to ask about Jim.' Here it is clear that much shared experience is being drawn upon so that despite the conversational style, the reader will understand the nuances of the writing where no one else would. However, in the same letter, if we suppose that the writer were giving directions so that the reader could visit, the tone would be different, perhaps something like 'Turn left at the crossroads, take the third on the right, walk a hundred yards until you come to a white house with a green door . . .'. The writer will realize intuitively that to retain the previous style would make the writing confusing and less effective. Even the most everyday communication, for example a note to a tradesperson, needs to be written in an appropriate style.

The therapist will have many writing tasks to fulfil during the course of a working week, each of which may require a different style. These tasks may include the writing of case notes, written instructions for a patient to take home, a letter to a general practitioner and a student assessment. The therapist may be engaged in further study and have an essay due, or a research project to be written up. A notice may need to be written for the waiting room requesting patients to close the door. All this writing must be effective but each document will have a different style according to its purpose and the readers for whom it is intended.

The notice for the waiting room door, for example, might have the direct and no-nonsense approach 'shut the door', though this might strike the reader as impolite or authoritarian. A more persuasive and egalitarian tone might be 'We'll all be warmer if the door is kept shut', but the reader may find this patronizing. An appeal to better natures is contained in 'Please shut the door, the NHS needs to save every penny', but even this might be thought to carry an implicit political message. It might be better to use the strictly formal 'Patients are requested to shut the door when entering or leaving the waiting room.'

The therapist might want to write some instructions for a patient who needs to continue exercises at home after discharge from therapy, but who requires reminders about how to peform them correctly. Writing effective instructions can be difficult. What if, for example, a therapist wrote the following instructions?

(1) Stand with your feet astride leaning slightly forward.
(2) Allow your arm to hang down loosely in front of you, and swing your arm across your body and out to the other side.
(3) Maintaining the same standing position, circumduct your arm in front of your body, first in one direction and then in the other.
(4) Be sure that your arm is limp and relaxed before doing these exercises.
(5) Now put one foot in front of the other, as if you were about to walk, and swing your arm backwards and forwards.
(6) Do these exercises twenty times each.

These instructions avoid difficult language and jargon, except for the term 'circumduct' which the patient is unlikely to understand. It would also be more sensible to instruct the patient to relax (instruction 4) before commencing the exercises. It is unclear from these instructions how often the exercises should be performed: should they be done twenty times an hour, twenty times a day or twenty times a week? With these, as with many other instructions, diagrams would almost certainly assist in making the meaning clear.

Therapists need to use another style when writing assessments of students following a clinical placement. This kind of writing has more permanence than those previously discussed. The readership becomes more diverse and the contents will need to be supported and justified. What is written may be scrutinized by senior colleagues in the department, and read by the student who is the subject of the assessment. It will also be seen by the student's tutors in college and will thereby provide not only information about the student, but also an impression of the therapy department in which the student has been placed. In addition the assessment document will, no doubt, be referred to later when other assessments are made. Although it is clear that the same information needs to be passed to each of these parties, the therapist might prefer to write in a different style to each, but be unable to do so. Faced with the prospect of producing a piece of writing for such a diverse readership, many writers simply opt for phrases that are the equivalent of 'fair', 'could try harder' and 'a satisfactory term's work'.

It may be the case, for example, that a therapist feels that a student has, by and large, the makings of a good practitioner but may need some help and practice in one or two areas. Perhaps the student could be more patient and communicative with clients. Obviously, the student's tutors will need to be aware of this, but if, in the therapists's view, the reason for this behaviour is lack of self-confidence, then the therapist may be loath to write down anything which could further diminish the student's self-image. 'This student sometimes shows impatience with clients', might be fine for the tutors, but perhaps, something like 'This student needs to allow clients to set the pace of their own treatment rather more than at present' might be more useful to the student, even though it is less direct.

In institutions where assessments and reports are open to those about whom they are written, writers frequently develop codes and jargon to conceal their meaning, but over time even this becomes understood by readers. On school reports, for example, everyone knows that 'Could try harder' means that the pupil is hardly trying at all. Perhaps the language of patients' notes will change in a similar way now that patients have gained access to them.

Cultural diversity

As well as making careful choices regarding vocabulary and style, it is also necessary for writers to reflect on the shared or diverse cultural experiences between themselves and their readers. Readers understand writing within a personal context of age, class, religion, politics, economic position and so on. The more conscious writers are of cultural diversity, the more effective their writing will become. This position is neatly summed up by Elbow who states: 'Not paying enough attention to your audience is a problem inherent in the nature of writing itself' (1981: 177).

Conclusion

This chapter has attempted to explain how complex a procedure writing is, as indeed are all language processes. The writer is faced with the task of bringing together composite elements, such as vocabulary, grammar, tone and content, to form a meaningful whole, with due regard to the underlying purposes of the writing and its intended readership. However, it is hoped that the impression has not been gained that this is a near impossible feat to accomplish. Like any other constructive human endeavour, writing is worth doing well, and the skills required for this are within the grasp of any therapist. It is hoped that the remainder of this book will assist in the acquisition of these skills.

2

The Process of Writing

People write for many reasons; they may want to make money, get promotion, see their work in print, pass through a course successfully or share their ideas. Writing may be a hobby, a form of therapy, an aspect of their work or something pursued through a love of words. Whatever your motivation may be, and however ambitious your aims, you do not have to be a genius, or even unusually talented, to write and to publish your work.

There is a great deal of mystique surrounding the art of writing and the process of getting published. The belief is that it is something only 'they' can do. This is probably because most people rarely have the opportunity to see writers at work, so the struggles they go through to find the right word or phrase or to organize their material coherently are hidden from view. Kerton reminds us that anyone who is not illiterate can write, and that 'if you have something to say and you can transfer those thoughts from brain to paper, then you're in business' (1986: 4). It would, however, be misleading to pretend that writing is an easy task which requires no effort. What characteristics and abilities, then, does the therapist need to be a successful writer?

Who makes a good writer?

First and foremost, writing to a high standard is hard work: most writers prepare numerous drafts before their writing even begins to approach the standard necessary for publication. Reaching this standard does not require brilliance, but much more mundane characteristics like stamina and perseverance. Writing is also a time-consuming occupation, so although it can be done in almost any location, the necessary time must be found. Having a deadline does help some people to work regularly and achieve their goals, but only if it does not cause them undue anxiety. Legat believes that:

> Professional writers don't rely on inspiration. There may be occasional flashes of insight, sudden brilliant ideas, experiences which give a new urge to write or suggest a different and exciting approach, and writers seize on them gratefully. But that's not the way the bulk of writing gets done.
> (Legat, 1986: 21)

Perseverance, regular work and a basic ability to string words together, are probably all that is needed to enjoy success as a writer; however, Legat (1986) believes that other characteristics and abilities may also help. These include imagination, a love of words, a professional attitude, life experience, self-confidence, self-criticism and a certain selfishness in carving out sufficient time to write. Writers may also need to surmount a certain degree of fear in exposing their ideas, and must be prepared to take risks.

Fear probably inhibits more people from publishing written material than anything else. Writing can seem to be fraught with risks because having one's ideas published gives them a certain permanence which is not shared by the spoken word. Publishing your material also provides other people with insights into your attitudes and personality which might subsequently work against you, for example when applying for a job. Opening oneself to scrutiny does involve the risk of being criticized or ridiculed, but the risks should not be exaggerated.

Another fear that writers and potential writers may have, is that their ideas and attitudes will change, that they will later disagree with what they have published, or that they will view the issues from an entirely different angle. This fear rests upon the erroneous assumption that changing one's mind is wrong; yet nothing could be further from the truth. If we look back at our articles in a few years time and cringe, this will merely show that our thinking has developed. There is no need to feel that your ideas must be static, in fact it is very unlikely that you will find enough to write about if they are. Your writing may cause others to query their assumptions, to ponder upon your arguments and question the issues you have raised. If anyone disagrees with you strongly enough to let you know, be happy that they are sufficiently interested to read what you have written and to take it seriously.

Although possessing various abilities and characteristics is helpful to the writer, it should be emphasized that there is little to stop anyone who wants to write from doing so. As Hawthorne (1989) points out, writing can be done anywhere and at any time. Gender, age, class, where you live or whether or not you are disabled, are all completely irrelevant; indeed if there is something unusual in your personal biography, or your life has been particularly difficult, it may well provide a wealth of writing material. Qualifications, though sometimes helpful, are not necessary, and there are few start-up costs involved in writing. All you really need is a pen and paper and the motivation to get started. Legat (1991) believes that there is no better way of learning the craft of writing than actually practising it, and Cormack states: 'Although some help can be given to the beginner, there is no recipe which can ensure success, there is no easy route to producing high quality written material' (1984: 3). This chapter will focus upon writing articles for publication, but much of the information will apply equally well to other writing tasks such as essays, hand-outs, reports and books.

Finding ideas

Ideas can come from many different sources; you may get an idea from talking to someone, by overhearing a conversation in the waiting room, by reading, researching, seeing a picture, reading a quotation or from an experience you have had. If you are writing an essay or sitting an examination the original idea is likely to be someone else's; in one sense this can be a relief, but it can also make your task difficult. Although it is

not always easy to come up with a good idea, there is really
no shortage of material about which to write. Some writers
wonder whether they will run out of ideas, but they often
find that the more they write the more easily ideas seem to
come. Recently one of the authors (SF) had to teach 'group
dynamics' to a class of nurses who were undertaking a health
studies course. In the process of reading and making notes for
the lecture, a passing reference to the powerful influence of
minorities within groups was found. This prompted a small
literature search and, subsequently, an article on the topic.
You will find that the more you write, the more ideas you will
have, and the more astute you will become at recognizing the
makings of a good article. Some experienced writers become
very observant, to the extent of searching for an article in
almost everything they see and hear. Hines believes that:
'Article material is all around you, but you must learn to be
article conscious, to spot the germ of an idea, to cultivate it in
your mind, and if possible to find a new angle for it' (1987:
18).

Everyone has a great deal of experience which is worth
sharing; it does not have to be profound or unusual, just
interesting to other people. If something fascinates you, the
likelihood is it will fascinate others as well. Therapists are
increasingly expected to contribute to the professional literature; they all have valuable knowledge and experience which
is worth disseminating, and they are all potential contributors
at every stage of their careers. Students, for example, can be
encouraged and helped to reshape their course work for
publication.

Although it is very important to avoid plagiarism, it is
perfectly in order to expand on the ideas of others, to give
them a different perspective or to relate them to a different
situation. It is rare for academic writers to create something
entirely new. Wells (1986) suggests that we can ask 'Who?',
'What?', 'Why?', 'Where?', 'When?' and 'How?' about anything to generate ideas. He also warns us of the ephemeral
nature of ideas and advises us to write them down when they
arise. It is important that the ideas on which you base your
article capture your interest and motivate you to write.

It does, of course, help to be knowledgeable about the subject on which you intend to write, but it is not essential, as you can always search the necessary information out before you start. This comes as something of a revelation to many people who imagine that writers are great experts on all that they produce. This may be true of some, but certainly not all, and it is a great pity if such a belief inhibits you from writing. Some authors set themselves the task of writing an article in order to learn something new, and in this situation they are certainly not writing from a position of great knowledge or expertise, but rather, are setting themselves the goal of publishing an article as a way of motivating themselves to learn.

Whatever your method of finding ideas, it can be a great help to discuss them with your colleagues. This will help you to assess the value of your ideas, as well as clarifying your own thinking.

Gathering information

If you are writing from your own experience you will already have at your disposal the raw material of your article, but if you want to write an article of a more theoretical nature, or on a topic which is outside your experience, you will probably need to do some research. This may consist in reading around the subject, talking to a number of people, sending out questionnaires, carrying out some interviews or a combination of these and other methods. The search for information should be guided rather than random, and audio-visual sources of information should not be neglected. If research is needed a great deal of work occurs before you actually start to write.

When gathering information for your article, it is necessary to keep meticulous notes and to be very organized; nothing is worse than losing work or forgetting its source when you come to write it up. Organizing your references is particularly important, and it can take many hours and much hard work to trace them if they go astray: record them safely on a card index or on your computer. (See chapter 6 for more details on referencing).

Finding a structure

You will now be faced with a jumble of material, from many different sources, from which the content and order of your article, essay, hand-out or report must emerge. This is the point at which panic can so easily set in. There is often a feeling of being overwhelmed and a fear that the material can never be organized, but this need not be the case. Becker (1986) defines writing as an organizational act, which is an apt description at this stage, because what you need is not extraordinary talent, but a sensible system of organizing your material and the willingness to give the task the time it deserves. If you are writing solely from personal experience, you can make a good start by writing down everything you know on the topic. This brain-storming exercise will help to free your thinking and enable you to see the various themes that emerge and the ways in which they can be linked. Although you may have written down many ideas, the chances are that they relate to just a few major themes. Becker states that 'you can only learn how few thoughts you have, if you write them all down, set them side by side and compare them' (1986: 56). Already, the chaos begins to subside!

Your thoughts and ideas can then be physically arranged in non-linear patterns, such as a web. Figure 2.1 illustrates a web based on the topic of 'Stereotyping older people'. In this way you will see how your ideas relate to each other and how they can be ordered in your article.

It should be emphasized at this point that there is always more than one way of structuring a piece of writing, and there is rarely a best way; the writer is usually left with a choice, and often needs to compromise among various possibilities. Some ways of organizing material are technically and intellectually easier than others, and this may be a deciding factor. Some ideas may appear to fit nowhere and may ultimately need to be abandoned, but do not make choices like this too

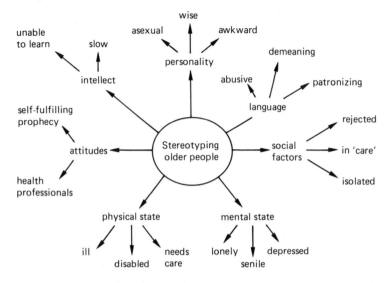

Figure 2.1   *Web based on the topic of 'Stereotyping older people'*

soon; when your article begins to take shape you may well see creative ways of weaving the ideas in.

If your writing is to be based on research material or notes which you have made, your organizational task is more laborious. One method, favoured by some authors, is to read carefully through all the material collected and give each point expressed a labelled number. For example when writing about pain perception and behaviour, number 1 could refer to 'the social context', number 2 to 'personality factors', number 3 to 'family attitudes and behaviour' and number 4 to 'past medical experiences'. A line can then be marked down the left hand side of the paragraph or section expressing the idea and a number written in the margin beside it. Then, on a separate sheet of paper, a list should be kept indicating to what the numbers refer. This is illustrated in Figure 2.2. When going through the material for the present chapter, the list included 'writers' characteristics', 'the use of punctuation', 'titles' and 'final draft'; in the end there were thirty-one points on the list. If reading has been extensive there is likely to be

1.	People may not feel very much pain if their attention is directed elsewhere, for example surviving in battle or competing on a sports field.
2.	Introverted individuals have been found by some researchers to have a lower pain threshold then extroverted individuals.
3.	Pain perception and behaviour is influenced by the behaviour and attitudes of family members.
4.	A painful visit to the dentist may heighten pain perception on a future visit.
2.	Research on personality factors in pain perception and pain behaviour conflicts.

1. The social context
2. Personallty factors
3. Family attitudes and behaviour
4. Past medical experiences

Figure 2.2 *Suggested way of organizing material*

repetition in your notes, so some material may need to be discarded. Do not feel concerned about this, the extra work will not have been wasted as it is likely to have equipped you with a sounder grasp of the subject.

Having categorized the material, the next task is to group the ideas into themes, which will often number about six, and then to work out, by means of non-linear thought patterns such as a web or flow-chart, how the themes can be structured within the article. Becker (1986) suggests that writers should use a system of cards to help them to organize their material at this stage. Each idea or point can be written on a separate card, and the cards then piled into themes, with the theme's heading written on the top one. The cards can then be arranged in various patterns indicating how the article could be structured. Becker is of the opinion that the greatest virtue of doing this is that it transfers a difficult mental task into a much simpler physical task. Having done this the task of writing can begin.

This all sounds very logical and precise, but to be quite truthful, some of us are impatient writers who rarely complete this process of planning before actually starting to write. We very often get stuck with too much thinking, and find that getting on with the writing loosens up our thoughts. You may find, for example, that you discover one or two major themes and start work on them right away without worrying about where all the other information will fit. It is quite in order even to start writing before you have finished the necessary reading and researching. Starting to write can clarify your thoughts concerning what else you need to read. All writers must organize their material, but the precise way in which they do so is to some degree idiosyncratic, and really does not matter as new information can be inserted at any stage.

Although you need some sense of direction before you start writing, it is not necessary to know exactly where the article is going or to have everything planned out in advance, neither does it matter if you never know all the answers to the questions you raise. The task of organizing your material has to be undertaken, but precisely how it is done is up to you. Starting a new article before the old one is complete can also maintain interest by providing variety; many writers like to have several pieces of work 'on the go' at once for this very reason.

Writing early drafts

Hines (1987) believes that the greatest hurdle for most beginners is getting their first few words down on paper. One reason for this may be that they feel they should start at the beginning. In fact the beginning is probably the most difficult place to start writing because, as Becker (1986) points out, writing is about thinking and learning and it is impossible to introduce a subject until you know exactly what it will concern. The introduction is, in fact, frequently written last. It is often worth starting with the areas you find easiest; by starting to write, some of the material is cleared, your thoughts are elucidated, you will feel more confident, and you may then feel able to tackle those parts which at first seemed quite beyond you. Start wherever it is easiest for you and never wait for inspiration; probably the best answer to procrastination and 'writer's block' is setting aside a regular time to write and sticking to it.

Your first draft should really be regarded as a voyage of discovery. There is no need to worry unduly about your grammar, spelling or phraseology at this stage. Do not be too concerned about how things sound or the crudeness of your draft, for it is important to realize that the first draft bears little resemblance to the one that will finally be sent to the editor or handed in for assessment. Keep in mind that you will write many more drafts and will be highly critical and meticulous later. If you get stuck, simply leave a little message to yourself in brackets, and come back to it later. In all probability the problems will sort themselves out as you progress with other areas.

It is a great advantage if a friend or colleague, knowledgeable about your chosen topic, or a sample of people representative of your potential readers, can be persuaded to comment on an early draft. Many of us have perfectionist tendencies which make it difficult to show someone such a rough document, but it really is worth while to get feedback at an early stage. It is unfortunate that people feel ashamed of their early drafts; a student in Becker's writing class always wrote on the second sheet of her pad so that she could quickly pull the top one down if anyone came near! Many of us can identify with these feelings, but if time is spent attending to detail early on, new ideas and insights may be stifled, and if a great deal of work is put in at this stage inhibitions about making necessary changes can build up. This having been said, some writers do edit their work as they go along; again, there are no hard and fast rules.

As you progress to later drafts, your alterations will become numerous and your document will look such a mess, that the very real danger of misunderstanding it yourself and getting confused will arise. Many writers work on A4 sheets of paper, writing on every second or third line to give themselves space for alterations. Even then, their work often gets so cluttered with corrections that a rewrite becomes essential, especially if someone else is being asked to type it up. Many writers now use word processors, but others simply use a system of 'stars' for inserting material into existing work. Thus if they want to insert a paragraph into their text, they write '*1' at the appropriate place in the text, as well as on the new paragraph or section to be inserted. There may in the end be very many stars for the typist to contend with, making clarity absolutely vital. Indeed, even if you type your own work, the same clarity is needed.

Some writers prefer to 'cut and stick'; if they find a paragraph which they believe would be better placed elsewhere in the text, they literally cut it out and stick it where it needs to go. For this method to work it is essential that one side of the paper is left blank. With a word processor, words and paragraphs can be moved, added and deleted at the press of a key, which makes revisions less laborious; the actual process is, however, exactly the same, and many people still prefer to write with no more equipment than paper and pen. Whatever system you use, it is good practice to preserve early drafts for reference.

Writing later drafts

When you are satisfied with the basic structure and content of your article or essay, the time has come to revise it, though, as noted earlier, many people prefer to revise as they go along. Do not be discouraged by the length of time revising takes, and remember that most professional writers spend a great deal of time pruning and perfecting their work. It helps to listen actively to what you have written, to hear those awkward words and clumsy phrases; so read your work aloud.

If you feel a little insecure about the accuracy of anything you have said, now is the time to check. It is also a good idea to confirm that you really understand the meaning of every word you have used. Be wary of similar words with significantly different meanings, look out for ambiguities in your writing and places where you have assumed the readers have background information they may lack.

Your writing must be very clear and as simple as possible for, unlike speaking with someone, there is no way of sorting out ambiguities and points of confusion. As a general rule, if you have used a word which had to be looked up in the dictionary, or one of which you have only recently learned the meaning, it may be wise to try to find a simpler one. If readers do not understand, it is usually the writer's fault rather than their own. Avoid using phrases from a foreign language, or abbreviations with which people may be unfamiliar or which may have more than one meaning. Double negatives, such as 'do not do this exercise if you are not feeling comfortable' or 'do not fail to take adequate precautions' are confusing and should be avoided. Above all, never attempt to sound clever or impressive. Your readership, and the purpose of your article, will determine your style and whether or not it is appropriate to use jargon and technical language; make all appropriate adjustments bearing these factors in mind.

This shaping and polishing process will involve considerable cutting. Every word should do some work and none should be wasted. Legat advises writers to 'cut anything which can come out without in any way damaging the impact of what you have written or the main points which you need to get across to the reader' (1986: 58). This includes the cutting of unnecessary adverbs and adjectives, explanations of the self-evident, words or phrases used solely out of habit, details which are unnecessary and repetition, unless this is done purposely for emphasis. Alternative words can be found if the same ones are repeatedly used (a thesaurus is invaluable here), and tired clichés, for example 'putting your back into it' or 'standing on your own two feet', should be avoided.

Redundant words (tautology), as in 'the patient continues to have *ongoing* problems with phonation' should be removed, and spelling should be checked. A good dictionary is essential to every writer, although many word processors have a facility for checking spelling. Punctuation will also need attention. By reading your work aloud the length of pause required can often be heard and will indicate whether you need a comma, semi-colon, colon or full stop. If you find it difficult to punctuate a sentence, it is probably too long. Underlining, exclamation marks, bold print and italics should all be used sparingly, since your writing should be sufficiently expressive to indicate where points of emphasis lie. On the whole, sentences and paragraphs should not be too long but should, nonetheless, vary in length to help give your writing rhythm and keep the reader interested. Several different points should not be made in the same paragraph, but long paragraphs expressing just one point can be divided. This pruning and cutting often leaves theoretical muddles and ambiguities exposed, so even at this late stage ideas can be developed and made more explicit.

Do not forget your readers at this stage; anticipate their difficulties and try to ensure that your writing is stimulating and that your argument progresses logically from one point to the next. Lewis (1979) points out that muddled writing usually results from muddled thinking. Although it is important that your writing is concise, Barrass (1982) warns that it should not be so dense that readers have insufficient time to grasp one point before the next one is presented. If your readers become confused, they are very likely to stop reading and toss your work aside; Whale (1984) believes that we should never knowingly oblige a reader to read the same sentence twice. In general try to be concrete rather than abstract, but if abstract concepts are discussed back them up if possible with concrete examples, ensuring that the examples really fit what you are trying to explain and do not merely serve to distract the reader from the main argument.

Quotations can be used to provide variety and to indicate that others agree with your views, but quoting should not be overdone and should be integrated with your own ideas and interpretations. Metaphors can liven up your work, but they must be fresh or they become clichés. Careless metaphors can also give rise to the wrong images which, far from enhancing your meaning, only serve to distract and confuse the reader.

Most writers have a tendency to write too much. More is not necessarily better, but it is no bad thing if your drafts are longer than required, because you then have the opportunity to select the material which suits your purpose best. Do not discard unwanted material too readily though, as it could well form the basis of your next piece of work. You may, on the other hand, find that certain parts of your work lack substance and need to be expanded. Do not be discouraged if you conclude that virtually the whole draft needs to be rewritten, this is quite normal and should give no cause for alarm.

Make sure that your opening paragraph catches the reader's attention; it should be interesting, or even controversial, so that the reader is induced to go on. Sometimes an interesting quotation can be used to open an article. The body of the article should consist of paragraphs which link your arguments logically and coherently into various themes. Great efforts should be made by the writer to ensure that the reader does not lose the thread of what is being said. Headings and sub-headings can help to break up the text and to make your meaning and the flow of ideas clear.

The conclusion is often difficult to write. It may simply recapitulate what has gone before, draw the main points of the article together or remind readers of the purpose of the article. It may give direction as to future developments, spell out the objectives the readers should now be equipped to achieve, give the ideas a new emphasis or place them in a different perspective. Articles sometimes end with an apt quotation. The ending must be satisfying and not leave the reader with the sense of being let down or confused, although conclusions which end with a thought-provoking comment can be very effective. Wells (1983) advises writers to end with 'a bang', just as they began.

Finding a suitable title for an article can be very difficult and is often the final task rather than the first. There is certainly no need to worry if you cannot think of one at the beginning. Ideally titles should catch people's attention and tempt them to read. Witty, sensational or controversial titles are all ideal, but simple, straightforward ones can be effective too. Wells (1983) suggests that titles fall into six broad types. Firstly, there is 'the label' which clearly states what the article is about, then there is 'the question' which can be linked to a provocative statement, for example 'Are Therapists Worth The Money? – Administrators at Clanford Hospital Think Not'. The title can also be in the form of a quotation, for example 'Lies, Damn Lies and Statistics' for an article on government health expenditure, or a twisted quotation, as in 'What Cannot be Cured Need Not be Endured'. Other types mentioned by Wells are those in the form of an exclamatory statement, such as 'Why I resigned as District Speech and Language Therapist' and those in the form of a pun, for example 'Striking Therapists Flex Their Muscles'.

Sometimes editors change the title of an article, only to give a false impression of what it is about. One of the present authors entitled an article on the placebo effect 'The Powerful Placebo', boring perhaps, but nevertheless reflecting its content. The editor changed the title to 'Magic Pills' which was more eye-catching but failed to reflect the content of the article, especially as its major aim was to demystify the placebo effect. On another occasion, an article written after carrying out some research, was entitled by the editor, 'Obesity – a Greater Stigma than Disability'. Certainly eye-catching and even sensational, but in the light of the findings in question this was not a central issue. The less academic the newspaper or journal, the more editors are liable to change the title and content of your work. They are skilful people and the result is as often pleasing as not. (Special care is needed when choosing a title for a research report, as explained in chapter 7.)

After reading and re-reading your own work many times you may become conditioned to it and less critical of it than you might otherwise be; you may not realize that the phrase you chose so carefully is ambiguous or that such a lengthy explanation of a point is unnecessary. There are two ways of dealing with this. You can put your work away for a few days or weeks and then re-read it, by which time you will be more detached and able to view it in a different light. Alternatively, you can give it to somebody else to read who is prepared to be critical. Someone used to dealing with written language, such as a teacher, is ideal. Some writers adopt the policy of trying their work out on someone who has no specific expertise in the area concerned, as an indication of its comprehensibility. Although this is a useful strategy, it will not work with all subject areas, for example those which are highly technical.

After so much pruning and feedback you will need to tidy up your article and ensure it still makes sense. If your work is for publication, editors will always prefer that which needs the least attention, and if you can achieve a high standard, you may be asked to write for the journal again.

Another task is to select tables, pictures, photographs and diagrams if you feel they will enhance your writing. This will be discussed in detail in chapter 8, but suffice it to say at this point that this task may occur before your writing is complete; indeed pictures, tables and diagrams may be the central focus of your article, rather than merely providing support for what you have written.

If you are writing a book, you may also need to write a preface or introduction, acknowledgements, a dedication, a contents list, tables and diagrams, a glossary, a bibliography and an index. Needless to say these should be written with just as much care. Cormack (1984) believes that although there is no such thing as a perfect manuscript, we all have the responsibility to write as well as we are able.

Conclusion

According to Lewis (1979) writing involves having something to say and having the ability and the confidence to write it down. Writing takes time and patience, perseverance and mental stamina. It does not, however, require extraordinary talent, creativity or expertise and is something every therapist can do. Hines states:

> It would be true to say that no writer ever masters his craft. He improves, of course, but perfection in writing is unattainable. Most of us will never reach great heights, it must suffice to do our best and constantly try to improve.
>
> (Hines, 1990: 125)

3

Avoiding Language which Stereotypes People

Many people are of the opinion that language should not be changed and that grammatical rules and conventions, such as putting 'he' before 'she', are sacred and immovable. In reality language constantly evolves as the meaning of some words changes, other words become obsolete and new words are invented. The word 'man', for example, has now largely narrowed to mean 'a male human being', whereas before the eighteenth century it referred to both males and females.

Our attitudes towards words can also change, an example of this is the word 'black' when referring to an Afro-Caribbean person; this used to be regarded as offensive, but is now used by many Afro-Caribbeans, as well as people from other ethnic minorities, as a symbol of solidarity and pride. Similarly, deaf people have reclaimed the word 'deaf' as a positive, rather than a negative, label.

Different groups within society have unequal power when it comes to challenging, shaping and changing language. Standard language reflects the prejudices of the more power-ful sections of society and has been used as a way of oppressing others. Thus women, old people, people from ethnic minorities and disabled people, who lack this power, have consistently been described in inaccurate and demeaning ways which have undervalued them and set limits on their lives. The term 'working mother', for example, implies that being a mother does not involve real work, and the over-use of the word 'care', when talking of old and disabled people, has no doubt played its part in fostering false images of dependency. By taking seriously the ways in which people are described and defined, we are not merely engaging in semantic games, for these definitions often form the basis upon which policy is made, services planned and delivered and resources allocated.

Some people find it hard to believe that language has such a powerful influence on our attitudes and behaviour, and may find the struggles people are engaged in to change terminology which they find offensive or inaccurate, rather trivial – the women's movement has certainly suffered its fair share of ridicule in this regard. There can, however, be no doubt that our attitudes are reflected in the language we use and are shaped by the language we hear (Spender, 1985).

It is well known by linguists and anthropologists that people from different cultures view the world, at least in part, according to the language they use and the way they categorize objects and people, for language is by far the most powerful means we have of shaping and sharing our thoughts and ideas. When British Rail decided to call us 'customers' rather than 'passengers' we may have considered it little short of a joke, but nonetheless, such changes of terminology have the potential to influence the attitudes of both railway staff and ourselves, for unlike the passenger, the 'customer is always right'. Reality is thus constructed through talk, and those who control talk control reality (Spender, 1985).

Many writers now strive to avoid sexist, racist, ageist and disablist language in their writings. This is not an easy task as the negative attitudes towards these groups of people are deeply embedded within our language and within society. Sometimes people are inhibited about changing the way they express themselves in writing, whatever their beliefs, because change can sound odd, clumsy and incorrect. It is always helpful to remember that many of the ways in which we express ourselves are relatively modern and that what may seem a radical change can soon become accepted. Examples of such changes are 'chairperson' rather than 'chairman', 'parenting' rather than 'mothering' and 'Down's Syndrome' rather than the offensive term 'mongolism'. If enough people with adequate power feel sufficiently strongly that a change in language is necessary, it will occur.

Avoiding sexist language

Sexist language can be defined as language which stereotypes on the basis of sex. Although both sexes are implicated, most of the negative stereotypes are directed at women.

Perhaps the most obvious problem any writer trying to avoid sexist language encounters, is which personal pronoun to use. If we do not know the sex of the person to whom we are referring it is a convention to use 'he', 'him' or 'his', rather than 'she', 'her' or 'hers'. Thus most people would write 'Do not bombard the patient with questions before *he* has had a chance to explain *his* symptoms', rather than 'Do not bombard the patient with questions before *she* has had a chance to explain *her* symptoms'. It is interesting to note that this custom did not appear until the eighteenth century; it is currently being widely challenged.

In everyday speech we tend to use 'they', 'their' and 'them' when we do not know the sex of the person concerned; thus our sentence becomes, 'Do not bombard the patient with questions before *they* have had a chance to explain *their* symptoms'. This is grammatically incorrect because 'the patient' is singular and 'they' and 'their' are plural, but people do express themselves in this way when speaking, and most do so when writing until they are corrected. In view of this many people feel it is rather pedantic to insist on 'correct' grammar when it does not convey the meaning adequately, and many writers ignore this rule.

Other writers get round the personal pronoun problem by using double pronouns i.e. he/she or s/he. This is, of course, non-sexist, but does tend to be awkward and clumsy if used too frequently. Another way of solving the problem is to use 'she' on some occasions and 'he' on others. This can work well but does have the potential to be confusing unless great care is taken. When writing in a relatively informal style, the word 'you' can be used instead of 'he' or 'she'. Thus rather than saying 'Before doing the exercise *he* should relax', the sentence could read, 'Before doing the exercise *you* should relax' or, in more formal writing, 'Before doing the exercise *one* should relax.' A further way of solving this problem is to eliminate personal pronouns altogether. Thus the above sentence could become, 'It is important to relax before doing the exercise', or the sentence can be made plural as in, 'People should relax before they do the exercise.'

Language which is demeaning to particular groups of people should always be avoided. There are many blatant examples of offensive and patronizing language directed at both women and men. One way of demeaning women is to focus on their physical attributes while, at the same time, focusing on the character or achievements of men. Language which focuses on incidental characteristics distracts the reader. An example of this would be: 'The eminent otolaryngologist Mr Smith, and the attractive speech and language therapist Miss Jones, both attended the conference.' One way of checking whether a sentence is sexist is to reverse the adjectives so that they refer to the person of the other sex. Thus our sentence would read: 'The handsome surgeon Mr Smith, and the eminent speech and language therapist Miss Jones, both attended the conference.' I think most people would agree that this sentence sounds inappropriate and even amusing.

Even if women's other attributes, such as their achievements, are acknowledged, it is common to mention their physical characteristics as well. An example might be: 'Miss Jones, the acclaimed and very attractive speech and language therapist, attended the conference in an elegant, blue, silk dress.' By mentioning the fact that Miss Jones is attractive and by describing the dress she wore to the conference, the reader's attention is distracted from her professional standing as a speech and language therapist. It also gives the covert message that professional standing and achievement are incompatible with beauty, or even with being a woman. A similar sentence referring to Mr Smith sounds entirely inappropriate – 'Mr Smith, the acclaimed and very handsome surgeon, attended the conference in a smart, blue, tailored suit.'

Merely mentioning a person's sex can be an irrelevance and a 'put-down': 'the prestigious, female consultant' or 'the famous, male nurse' give a subtle message that these people are non-standard and that their sex is incompatible with their occupation. It can also be confusing as we are left wondering whether the doctor is prestigious in terms of female doctors or all doctors, or whether the nurse is famous for his achievements as a nurse or as a male nurse.

As well as their physical characteristics, women's domestic responsibilities and family relationships are also mentioned far more often than those of men. Thus we have descriptions such as: 'The famous politician, housewife and mother of six, won the recent by-election.' The message here is either that becoming a politician is an extraordinary feat for a housewife and mother, or that housewives and mothers have no business being politicians. Similarly it is often assumed in written and spoken language that women are responsible for all domestic tasks. On the Radio 4 programme 'Farming Today' it is always the *housewife* who is alarmed at the price of tomatoes, perpetuating the view that it is the rôle of women, rather than men, to shop and cook.

Health professionals can also perpetuate these stereotypes in their writing. In a self-help booklet entitled 'Hysterectomy and Vaginal Repair' (Lobo and Taylor, 1988) examples of the activities people should and should not do following surgery are in terms of 'household duties', for example dusting, ironing and shopping, and the correct way of picking up heavy objects is illustrated by a woman lifting a laundry basket.

Character stereotyping should be avoided too. Men and women both display the full range of human characteristics, attributes and emotions, making words such as 'womanly' and 'manly' sexist, misleading and inaccurate. 'Manly' refers to strong, positive characteristics, such as 'bravery' and 'stoicism', whereas 'womanly' refers to both positive and negative characteristics such as 'fickle', 'irrational', 'gentle' and 'warm'. Even the positive characteristics assigned to women tend to be passive. This is not to imply that women cannot be fickle and irrational, of course; the point is that men can be too. The positive images assigned to men, such as confidence and strength, can also be oppressive as they force men to deny many aspects of their personalities, namely those typically assigned to women. Identical behaviour on the part of men and women is often referred to in different ways; with women's behaviour usually being regarded more negatively; thus whereas men 'debate' women 'bicker', and whereas men 'get angry' women have 'temper tantrums' or become 'hysterical'.

If women are likened to men it is usually regarded as a great compliment. Phrases such as: 'She's as good as any man in that job' or 'She's the one who wears the trousers', carry the message that she is very competent and not at all typical of women. If men are referred to as women, on the other hand, as in 'he's such an old woman', it is regarded as a great insult. (For more detail on avoiding sexist language, the reader is referred to Miller and Swift, 1989.)

Avoiding ageist language

The term 'ageism' was coined by Butler (1975) and can be defined as a process of systematic discrimination and stereotyping of people simply because of their age. No age group is exempt from age-related stereotypes; thus children may be viewed as unreliable, teenagers as irresponsible and middle-aged people as 'past it' by many potential employers. However, there can be no doubt that old people are affected by ageist attitudes more than any other age group and that these attitudes are reflected in our language.

Ageist language has much in common with sexist language. For example the language used to describe old people often insults, belittles and diminishes them. Knowles (1987) complains that it is not uncommon for nurses to refer to older patients as 'dear', 'darling', 'love', 'poppet' and 'sweetie', and believes that most old people find this patronizing and embarrassing. The tendency automatically to call old people by their first names, or by terms of endearment such as 'granny', are also demeaning, especially when the person using this language expects to be addressed in a more formal way. Even physical abuse of old people is trivialized by such expressions as 'granny abuse' and 'granny bashing' – terms which can be found in the professional literature.

Terms such as 'the elderly' and 'the aged' can also be criticized for fostering the impression that old people form a homogeneous group, whereas in reality they are as heterogeneous as any other large section of the population, even in terms of their age. Such language is also dehumanizing, indeed it is not uncommon for the person to be omitted altogether, as in the chapter heading 'Working with Abuse' (Pritchard, 1992: 41). Such dehumanizing language is not uncommon in employment advertisements for health professionals, as well as in their journals and textbooks.

The word 'care' has also been questioned as it fosters a dependent and helpless image which is usually quite inappropriate. Despite this the medical speciality 'care of the elderly' has now been adopted in favour of 'geriatrics', yet we do not talk about 'care of the young' or 'care of the middle aged'. It is interesting to note that the Open University course 'Caring for Older People' has been renamed 'Working with Older People'. The term 'geriatrics' was at one time neutral, referring to a medical speciality, like 'paediatrics' or 'orthopaedics', but took on such a derogatory character, because of the negative attitudes towards old people, that it has had to be abandoned.

The word 'old' is frequently used as a term of abuse, for example: 'old fool', 'old bag', 'old maid' and 'old dragon'. Old women are at a particular disadvantage as they are subject to both ageist and sexist stereotypes. The phrase 'being an old woman' is sexist as well as ageist as it implies that old women are particularly fussy and ineffective. The use of the word 'senile' as a synonym for dementia is also ageist as senile merely means 'relating to old age'. Terms such as 'dirty old man' and 'mutton dressed as lamb' indicate our distaste of any sexual activity among old people, and the adage that 'you can't teach an old dog new tricks' indicates the widespread and erroneous belief that old people are incapable of learning new skills. In reality people continue to learn effectively throughout their lives and many people remain sexually active into old age.

It is unfortunate that when old people achieve something, even something quite modest, they are frequently praised and congratulated simply because they are old. Thus we have descriptions such as 'Sprightly grandad, 75, walks marathon' or 'Incredible granny, 79, gains degree.' This type of writing perpetuates the misconception that old people are physically and mentally unfit and that the particular people being referred to are extraordinarily exceptional. The wording of these sentences would sound quite inappropriate in describing a younger person. Charities and the media have much to answer for in perpetuating ageist stereotypes. The person's age and relationships should not be mentioned unless they are strictly relevant.

Writers should avoid perpetuating personality stereotypes of old people: old people do, of course, have the same range of characteristics, attributes and emotions as everyone else. Most of the personality traits assigned to old people are negative and include lack of adaptability, forgetfulness, selfishness, stubbornness, awkwardness and inflexibility, to name just some. Even the few positive stereotypes assigned to old people, such as their supposed wisdom, are misleading and should be avoided. There is, in fact, no sharp discontinuity of personality with age, and what changes there are are usually a consequence of life experience or the result of the situation the person is in. Writers should avoid individualizing the behaviour of old people or the problems they may experience. For example old people who talk a lot about the past may do so, not because they are old, but because their present life lacks stimulation which, in turn, may result from lack of money or social facilities. Their behaviour may be perfectly rational when the situation they are in is taken into account.

Avoiding disablist language

Disablist language can be defined as language which stereotypes on the basis of disability or impairment. The terms 'disability', 'impairment' and 'handicap' tend to be used interchangeably. Organizations of disabled people (that is, those which are controlled by disabled people themselves) define impairment as bodily malfunction, for example inability to see, walk or hear, and disability as the limitations imposed upon the individual by the interaction between the impairment and the physical and social environment. Thus lack of braille and lack of accessible buildings are considered to create disability. The term 'handicap' is not used by organizations of disabled people, though it is used in certain classification systems such as that of the World Health Organization.

The words 'illness', 'disease', 'sickness' and 'disability' are often used interchangeably. This should be avoided as many disabled people are extremely fit and healthy, which is not to deny that disability and illness can, and frequently do, co-exist. Although there is no absolute consensus among disabled people concerning how they should be defined, it is recommended that writers define disabled people and disability in line with organizations *of* disabled people. Thus disability should be viewed largely as existing in the physical and social environment, rather than within disabled people themselves, and much thought should be given before the problems which disabled people encounter are portrayed as their personal problems.

Thought should also be given as to whether to use the word 'need' or 'right'. Basic human rights are often regarded as disabled people's needs, for example the need for an accessible toilet or the need for integrated education. The same can be said of old people. The translation of rights into needs depoliticizes disability.

Language which defines people in terms of their impairments should also be avoided, for example 'He's an amputee' or 'She's a hemiplegic.' This gives the impression that the impairment is the disabled person's most important attribute, and also tends to reduce the person to a medical condition. This type of criticism can also be levelled against terms such as 'the disabled' and 'the handicapped' which, as well as assuming that disabled people form a homogeneous group, defines them by one facet of their entirety. This having been said, some disabled people and their organizations deliberately use terms such as 'the blind', 'the deaf' and 'the disabled' as an expression of pride, strength and solidarity.

Alternative descriptions are 'disabled people' and 'people with disabilities'. Some people dislike the term 'disabled people' as they think it concentrates too much on disability at the expense of the person. Others believe that 'people with disabilities' should be avoided as it individualizes disability, depicting it as something disabled people *have* rather than something which is imposed on them by society. It can also trivialize the experience of disability which is usually a very central feature of the person's life. The preferred term among organizations *of* disabled people is 'disabled people' and it is recommended that writers use this term.

Many words give the impression that disabled people are dependent and helpless whereas, in reality, most live active and productive lives if given the opportunity to do so. The word 'disabled' (not able) and 'invalid' (not valid) illustrate this point. Words such as 'incurable' and 'infirm' should generally be avoided. The terms 'care' and 'caring for' should be used with caution; many disabled people prefer to use words like 'enable', 'assist' and 'working with'. Charities, in their efforts to arouse public sympathy and concern, and perhaps to perpetuate their own positions of power, have frequently portrayed a false and harmful image of disabled people as pitiable and in need of care. Images such as these have been portrayed, not only through words, but also through the use of logos.

There should be an emphasis on what people can do rather than on what they cannot do, and people who assist disabled people should not be viewed as saints and heroes as this portrays disabled people in very negative terms. On the other hand, it may be important to emphasize the very real stresses disabled people, and those who assist them, experience due to lack of social support. All of this is equally true of old people.

Language which depersonalizes should be avoided. This type of language is still commonly heard among health professionals and includes such terms as 'dealing with' disability and referring to people as 'cases'. Terms such as 'patient' and 'client' can give the impression that disabled people are in need of professional ministrations. 'Customer' and 'consumer' have been suggested as words which indicate greater equality, but there is always the danger of such words becoming mere euphemisms. Language which focuses excessively on the problems, limitations and difficulties of disabled people, and which perceives them as victims, should also be avoided. A delicate balance is needed here as writers may be keen to highlight the very real disadvantage experienced by many disabled people. This, however, should be balanced with accounts of the struggles disabled people are currently engaged in to remove structural and social barriers.

Abusive language should always be avoided. It is interesting that terms which were at one time used in a medical and legal context, for example 'idiot' and 'moron', have now taken on a derogatory meaning and are used as terms of abuse. Other abusive words, often to be heard in children's playgrounds, include 'cretin' and 'spastic'. Terms such as 'lame duck', 'deaf to reason', 'blind stupidity' and 'short-sighted' (meaning lacking insight) are commonplace in our language, showing how deeply embedded negative conceptions of disability are. Symptoms of illness or disability can also be used in this way, for example describing an irritating person as 'a pain' or using the word 'feeble' to describe an ineffective person. Other terminology tends to minimize disability, for example 'hard of hearing' rather than 'deaf' or 'partially deaf', and 'visually impaired' rather than 'blind'. Some disabled people (certainly a minority) prefer the word 'cripple' to 'motor impaired' as they believe it conveys a more accurate description of their situation.

Language which portrays disability as a personal tragedy should generally be avoided. This individualizes and depoliticizes disability and does not reflect the views of organizations of disabled people. Such terminology might include 'sufferers' and 'victims' and gives rise to notions of 'courage', 'bravery' and 'martyrdom' which most disabled people cannot identify with. Many people who acquire a disability do, however, talk of the personal anguish it causes them, and to ignore this is oppressive in itself. The equipment disabled people use should never be viewed negatively; few disabled people want to throw away their wheelchairs or walk. When writing about disability it is vital to consult disabled people themselves and to read what they have written.

Although the situation is beginning to change, disabled people are often portrayed either as helpless and pathetic or as superhuman. This can be seen very clearly in films, plays, novels and charity advertising. Disabled people also tend to be portrayed as asexual and as having unusual and mysterious gifts and powers, such as the sixth sense of the blind. This is not to deny that disabled people may develop certain skills because of the situation they are in, for example blind people may become very sensitive to echoes which help them to move about independently, but those sorts of abilities should never be portrayed as magic. Disabled people should be portrayed by writers as having the same range of attributes, emotions, desires, characteristics and aspirations as anyone else. If the language used would sound inappropriate when describing a non-disabled person, the chances are it is disablist.

Disability is also frequently portrayed in medicalized, individualistic terms with an overemphasis on cure which only serves to stress the conception of disability as tragic and unacceptable. Pictures and photographs of disabled people which are out of context and which focus on the person's impairment, are offensive to many disabled people. Images and stereotypes which appear positive can also have detrimental effects. For example if disabled people are always seen as being very capable it gives the impression that they do not need any help or consideration and saddles disabled people with the feeling that in order to be acceptable they must be superhuman. The unusual aspects of disability or impairment should not be overemphasized in an attempt to gain the reader's interest or to create variety. The curiosity and entertainment value of impairment and disability (and even the idea that it is an interesting subject) are offensive to many disabled people.

Avoiding racist language

Writers often become confused concerning which terminology to use when referring to people from ethnic minority groups. This is not surprising as there is little consensus among people from these ethnic groups themselves. Ahmad (1990) uses 'black' when referring to people from South Asian, African and Caribbean backgrounds, as well as other visible minority groups in Britain. She points out that the term is not used in order to depict these culturally diverse groups as homogeneous, but as a way of recognizing their united struggle against racism and discrimination.

Baxter (1988) defines Afro-Caribbeans as people born in the Caribbean Islands and their descendants. It is a rejection of the former term 'West Indian', which Afro-Caribbean people regard as a construct of British imperialism. She refers to Asians as people born in India or Pakistan and their descendants who were born in East Africa, as well as the British-born children of both these groups. Baxter et al. (1990) include people from Bangladesh and their descendants.

Baxter defines people from ethnic minority groups as members of minority racial groups, and an ethnic group as: 'a group of people who have certain background characteristics in common such as language, culture and religion, which provide the group with a distinct identity as seen both by themselves and by others' (1988: 2). The term, strictly speaking, covers white ethnic groups, such as people from Ireland and Scotland, but has really become a euphemism for 'black'. Terms such as 'ethnic people' and 'ethnic families' are meaningless; Baxter (1988) suggests that the terms 'ethnic minority' and 'ethnic majority' should be used.

The terms 'multiracial', 'multiethnic' and 'multicultural' tend to be used interchangeably. However, the term 'multicultural' implies that inequalities are brought about by our lack of understanding of cultural differences, and that all we have to do to eliminate such inequalities is to work at understanding each other better. Many people from ethnic minority groups object to the term as it denies the importance of racism in creating prejudice, discrimination and disadvantage.

Racist language can be defined as language which stereotypes people on the basis of race. It has much in common with sexist, ageist and disablist language. Many writers now take steps to avoid it, but racist language is still rife, particularly in the tabloid newspapers (Gordon and Rosenberg, 1989). People from ethnic minority groups are often portrayed, in spoken and written language, as social *problems*. Expressions such as 'the race *problem*' and 'the immigration *problem*' are common. People from ethnic minority groups, particularly young Afro-Caribbeans, are frequently portrayed as scroungers and law breakers, and there is extensive, exaggerated and distorted coverage of these issues in the press. The language which is used to describe these 'problems' is often provocative: refugees *flood* into Britain, Britain is *swamped* with immigrants and black people *rampage* in the streets. The fact that most immigrants in Britain are white is rarely mentioned. When people talk or write about 'Britain' they usually mean *white* Britain. Even though the majority of people from the ethnic minorities were born in Britain, they are rarely regarded as British.

People from ethnic minority groups are, in many ways, in a similar situation to people from other marginalized groups. Offensive terms, such as 'coloured' and 'half-caste', though once commonplace in everyday language, are no longer acceptable, and have been replaced by 'black' and 'mixed race'. Even the word 'immigrant' is frequently used in an abusive way. People from these groups are patronizingly overpraised for minor achievements, as if few others like them could achieve so much, and their ethnic origin is frequently referred to unnecessarily as in 'the brilliant black doctor'.

Gordon and Rosenberg (1989) point out that when people from ethnic minority groups are highlighted for having 'done well', there is usually a covert message, that because they have been successful racism cannot exist, and that complaints about it are merely an excuse for idleness. They are generally regarded as being less able than the majority population, just as women, old people and disabled people are. People write about the 'problems' of those from ethnic minority groups without consulting them, with the consequence that their needs are distorted, or their very existence denied, when services are planned and delivered.

It is important for writers to avoid personality stereotyping of people from these ethnic groups. Although some of these stereotypes appear to be positive, on the surface at least, for example 'hardworking Asians', most are negative and are frequently very mixed and almost contradictory. For example Afro-Caribbean people are portrayed as outgoing, violent and aggressive, but also as incapable, unintelligent and in need of authoritarian guidance.

Conclusion

Other groups of people who are subject to adverse stereotyping in written and spoken language could have been included in this chapter if space had allowed, for example people who are mentally ill, people with AIDS and those who are gay or lesbian. Much of what has been said will apply to these people too, although no oppressed group is ever identical to another in the prejudice and discrimination it experiences, so writers must become informed. All writers can play their part, however small, in helping to eliminate erroneous stereotypes which limit and oppress disadvantaged groups, and it is hoped that some of the suggestions in this chapter (for that is all they are) will be useful to therapists who are keen to write without stereotyping people.

Chapter

4

The Student Writer

Many students feel daunted by the writing tasks they must achieve. When they write they are often attempting to convey difficult concepts and ideas which have only recently been grasped and have yet to be fully assimilated. Essays, examinations and projects, which will be commented upon, criticized and assessed, can also cause stress and anxiety. This is understandable because written work usually plays a large part in the assessment process. As Barrass states: 'In any subject if students are equal in ability and intelligence those who are able to convey their thoughts clearly in writing will get the better marks' (1982: 1).

A problem often experienced by students, particularly at the onset of a course, is their unfamiliarity with the nature of the writing assignments required of them. Their recently completed school studies may leave them ill-equipped to write a research report, a lengthy project, or a clinical case study. Some students may have been away from formal education for some years, and may be coming to college after spending time bringing up a family or working in another field. While these experiences are likely to furnish students with many useful talents, as well as wide experience, writing may be a neglected skill or one which remains underdeveloped.

When studying at college you will frequently be writing for several readers at once. Completed essays, for example, may be useful to you when you come to revise, but they may also be scrutinized by several tutors who, in a real or imagined sense, have individual preferences. At the same time, if the work is part of your continuous assessment, it will be written with an examiner in mind; even if the tutor and the examiner are one and the same person, as is often the case in higher education, he or she will be performing dissimilar rôles which will give rise to different expectations.

Writing for several people at once can be complicated, but bearing a readership 'hierarchy' in mind will help. You should ask who has first need of any document you produce. Hospital notes, for example, which will remain *in situ* long after the clinical placement is over, should conform to the system in use, and examination answers should be written with the examiner in mind. Lecture notes, on the other hand, can be constructed entirely as best pleases you, whatever advice you are given.

Whatever you are asked to write, constraints will be placed upon you; indeed the tasks themselves are partly determined by the nature of these constraints. Essay writing, note-taking and coping with examination questions, for example, require rather different skills. In addition, you will usually be constrained by the number of words allowed, the materials and methods you may use, and the style of presentation, which varies according to the academic discipline.

This chapter will outline various approaches, strategies and processes which will help you to achieve your writing tasks and to overcome some of the difficulties you may encounter. It should be read in conjunction with chapter 2 'The Process of Writing', and chapter 8 'The Use of Graphics'. Writing research reports, which is dealt with in detail in chapter 7, will not be covered in this chapter.

Taking notes

Taking notes, from a lecture, from written material or from audio-visual sources, is often an important early step in the process of producing a piece of written work. Notes are made for three main reasons: to aid concentration, to aid understanding and creativity and to secure a record for the future (Rowntree, 1988). Notes express your own understandings, and if produced with care, are far more useful as an aid to learning, memory and revision than the sources from which they were made. Notes can be taken from any source, for example discussions, handouts, seminars and the ideas of peers; students sometimes form the erroneous belief that it is only worth taking notes from tutors.

It is important to keep the purpose of the notes in mind as this will determine the form they take. The notes may be needed later for revision, they may be used to construct a handout or report, or simply to jot down a few key words and apt quotations. Whatever the purpose of the notes may be, their usefulness will depend on your skill and efficiency in making them. If notes have been made under difficult circumstances, for example from a tutor who was talking too fast, they will need to be rewritten without delay while the material still makes sense. Notes from tutors usually serve merely as an outline which needs to be added to later with materials from other sources. The form that lecture notes take is partly determined by the way tutors present their material.

Students sometimes have a tendency to copy whole passages of text word for word when making notes, rather than extracting the major points. They are unlikely to learn very much from this process. Writing notes will only aid your understanding and concentration if you are actively engaged in producing them, and if your notes are very long they will be unsuitable for revision purposes. In addition, placing pieces of other people's text verbatim in your own amounts to plagiarism which is never permissible, though it is perfectly in order to use the ideas of others and to quote from their work. A far more efficient and active way to learn is to précis the text and put it into your own words. Barrass (1982) advises students to make their notes concise, and once they have fully grasped the main points to go back and reduce them still further. Eventually the notes, which may once have covered several pages of A4 paper, may comfortably fit on a few record cards.

Rowntree (1988) distinguishes between 'taking' notes and 'making' notes. When notes are 'taken' students tend to copy large chunks of text or attempt to write down everything the tutor utters. 'Making' notes, on the other hand, is a far more active and creative process as students synthesize and modify the material as they put it into their own words. Copying notes from other students is not very useful; not only do students come to the subject with different levels of knowledge and understanding, making the content of their notes unsuitable for other people, but the active processes of assimilating and organizing the material are lost if notes are merely copied. Research generally supports the idea that note taking, and encoding the notes later, aids attention and understanding (Newble and Cannon, 1990).

There are various methods of making notes which vary according to their purpose and the individual preference of each student; there is no *correct* method. The three main approaches are:

(a) straight prose
(b) skeleton outlines
(c) patterned notes.

Lecture notes are rarely seen by other people and students are likely to benefit if tutors spend time advising them on taking notes. Brown and Atkins (1988) suggest that one way of raising awareness is for students to compare their notes in pairs or small groups and evaluate each other's strategies.

Straight prose

Notes of this type, sometimes referred to as sequential or linear notes, consist of a précis of the lecture or text. Provided it *is* a précis the notes should be useful, but 'rewriting the textbook', by copying large pieces of text verbatim, is too passive a process to be of much value; as Rowntree states: 'The essence of effective note-taking is selectivity' (Rowntree, 1988: 158).

Well-known abbreviations such as '<' for 'less than' can be used, as well as highlighting, underlining and various symbols which may be idiosyncratic and understood only by the student; a straight line in the margin may signify a particularly important point, a wavy line may distinguish your own thoughts from the lecture content, and an exclamation mark may highlight an area with which you disagree. A question mark may indicate a point you do not understand, and a cross that further work needs to be done. Various systems of colour coding can also be used. It is not a good idea to use shorthand or speed writing as this will encourage you to write everything down verbatim, which will inhibit the active learning process.

Skeleton outlines

It may be appropriate for you merely to record key words, brief phrases and further references. You may, for example, wish to avoid the examples which the tutor or textbook gives, preferring to provide your own, or you may already have considerable information on the topic in question and wish only to supplement your knowledge.

Patterned notes

These are two dimensional, non-linear notes which provide a flexible alternative to conventional note-making. The central idea of the lecture or text is placed in a box in the middle of the page, lines radiate out from the box and related concepts are placed at the end of each line. This process continues with lines projecting out from the secondary concepts in a web-like structure. Comments can be written on the lines to indicate the nature of the relationship between the various concepts. One of the advantages of patterned notes is that they will force you to select the most important points.

Suppose, for example, that a tutor begins a lecture on the subject of 'The therapist/patient relationship' thus:

> There are many areas in which the relationship between a therapist and a patient may run into difficulties. Firstly there may be social class and cultural differences between them, secondly there may be barriers created by their different levels of knowledge and expertise, and thirdly, there may be personal and social factors relating to the patient, which the therapist does not fully understand, or fails to take into account.

With conventional notes your notepad, by this stage, may look something like Figure 4.1:

The therapist/patient relationship
Three main areas where it may flounder:
    (1) Social class and cultural differences
    (2) Different levels of knowledge and expertise
    (3) Personal/social factors

Figure 4.1   *Information presented using conventional notes*

Whereas with the patterned notes it will look more like Figure 4.2:

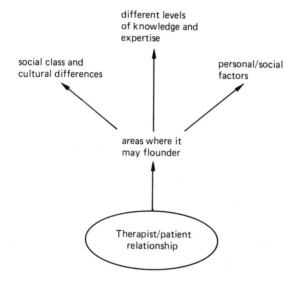

Figure 4.2   *Information presented using patterned notes*

The tutor may go on to expand on this theme as follows:

To enlarge upon my first point, differences in social class and culture may cause constraints between the therapist and the patient relating to race, gender and language.

With regard to their knowledge and expertise, the therapist is likely to have more detailed knowledge of disease processes, but the patient will know more than the therapist about the experience of his or her particular illness. There may be conflict between them concerning the meaning of symptoms.

To enlarge upon my third point, the patient may view the therapist as an authority figure and show undue deference as a result. The therapist will control the encounter in many ways, for example the timing, and may decide which treatment, if any, to give.

By this time, students writing linear notes may already be wondering how they can be disentangled later (see Figure 4.3).

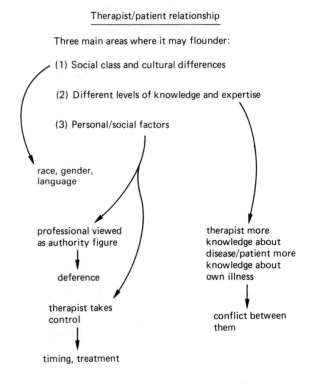

Figure 4.3   *Information presented using linear notes*

Whereas students using the patterned notes may still be retaining clarity (see Figure 4.4).

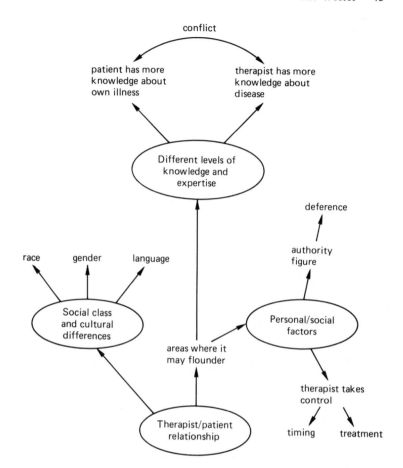

Figure 4.4   *Information presented using patterned notes*

Patterned notes are not without their limitations, however; Rowntree (1988) has found that they get a mixed reception. They force students to use very few words which may impede the expression of complex arguments, and information such as references cannot easily be included. In addition it is easy to run out of space and for the page to become overcrowded. Barrass (1984) believes that patterned notes are difficult to correct, amend or add to, and that they are unsuitable for subjects such as mathematics and science where the logical development of an argument must be recorded. They appear to work best with the social sciences and humanities where a clear hierarchy of ideas is less evident. Some students reserve this method for 'brain storming' before they start to write notes, others transform linear lecture notes into a web structure after the lecture, while others use a mixture of linear and patterned notes. Dunleavy (1986) advises that notes are a purely personal aid and that students should not feel constrained to use any particular format unless it suits their needs.

For further information on patterned notes, the reader is referred to Buzan (1989).

Writing essays

Writing essays is the written task most often demanded of students. A great deal of learning takes place when students write essays as it helps them to organize their thinking, explore topics in greater depth, reconstruct the ideas of others and clarify their own understandings. Effective essay writing promotes intellectual development, and its active nature helps students to internalize newly acquired knowledge. In this way it can assist students to défend and discuss their own opinions and ideas. Rowntree states: 'Writing is a crucial step without which learning is incomplete' (1988: 150). He believes that 'preparing essays should be seen as part of the learning process – not as a troublesome chore that follows it' (1988: 149).

As well as providing a valuable learning activity, essays give you practice in written communication and provide an important form of contact between you and your tutors. Your essays can indicate to tutors how far you have assimilated the material, and gives them an opportunity to make suggestions, provide you with encouragement, and supply feedback concerning errors, omissions and misunderstandings. Essays are also very useful for examination revision; it is vital never to hand one in without first taking a copy!

It is extremely important when writing an essay that you understand the question and answer it precisely. This is not to imply that only one answer is possible or correct, but to emphasize the importance of keeping the particular question being asked in mind. Underlining or highlighting key content and instruction words, and referring back to the question frequently, will help you not to stray from the question being asked. It is vital to look carefully at words which indicate *how* the question is to be answered. Being asked to *describe* requires a different response than being asked to *analyse critically* or *compare and contrast*.

There is a continuing debate in educational circles, and in the media generally, as to the importance of correct grammar, spelling and punctuation. Lack of skill in these areas, as well as poor presentation, may irritate and distract, but more importantly it can easily lead readers to become genuinely confused which may, in turn, adversely affect your grades. One way of avoiding grammatical mistakes is to read the finished text aloud where errors may be heard or, alternatively, to ask one or more people with the necessary skill to read it through and give you their comments. There are many books available to help you with grammar, spelling and correct English usage. A few of these will be listed under 'Bibliography' at the end of the book.

Students sometimes feel that they ought to use an 'academic' style. If this does not come naturally but rather feels remote and unfamiliar, then its use is unnecessary; it is far more important to write clearly and simply. Changes of style rarely happen speedily, but over years of writing within a given field, as knowledge is accumulated, a particular style may develop to suit specific needs or conform to professional norms. You should generally present material in a fairly detached tone, although some assignments may require you to be more personally involved. You may, for example, be asked to describe your feelings after visiting a hospice.

One of the main elements in essay writing is to demonstrate to the reader that recent publications and research, appropriate to the topic, have been read, understood and assimilated. These sources of information should be referenced correctly in an appropriate and consistent style. (For further discussion of referencing, the reader is referred to chapter 6.)

Essays should not be repetitive and padded with extraneous material, such as numerous examples illustrative of a single point. Repetition can give readers the impression of 'going round in circles' which does not aid understanding of what is being said. Statements should generally be supported by appropriate evidence, and speculative assertions should be made clear by using words such as 'possibly' or 'perhaps'. Essays should be balanced and well ordered, with each part receiving adequate thought and attention. The cardinal rule in essay writing is to refrain from anything which may result in loss of effective communication with the reader.

The best way of achieving a high quality essay is to plan it carefully before writing it. Barrass states that '[m]any students are clever enough to understand their work and yet unable to communicate their knowledge and ideas effectively' (1982: 4). Lewis (1979) believes that a thoughtfully constructed plan saves time, assists the student psychologically in writing the essay, and is more likely to result in a well-shaped product. Different types of written assignments require different plans; a plan for writing a physiological research report, for example, is likely to differ quite markedly from a plan preceding a sociology essay. (For detailed advice on planning and writing assignments, the reader is referred to chapter 2.)

It is important to work within the constraints of the essay writing task. The number of words allowed should be adhered to or time will be wasted and marks may be lost. If an essay, in the planning stage, looks as though it might be too long, it is likely that some of the information gathered is irrelevant or too detailed. If, on the other hand, it looks as though it might be too short, then important issues have probably been neglected. It is a good idea to discuss essay plans with tutors and fellow students.

The constraints of any writing assignment may be frustrating, but they can be used as a basis and discipline for developing various writing skills. Such skills may include the ability to express a complex idea, like illness behaviour, succinctly or in depth, to write about a single concept in depth, to use various styles for different readers, and to write fluently under the pressure of time.

Writing examinations

Many students find examinations the most difficult and stressful part of their assessment. In this situation there is little time for thought or planning and, with many examinations, reliance must be made on memory for all the information required. Even though every effort may have been made to learn and retain the knowledge demanded, an examination can still come as an unpleasant surprise. Thorough preparation and competent writing skills will, however, greatly enhance performance and reduce stressful feelings. A certain degree of anxiety is, however, advantageous as it stimulates and motivates us to achieve; it is only when it becomes too intense that our performance is adversely affected. The key to coping with examination writing is practice and experience. As Cormack states: 'As with all types of writing, answering examination questions requires not only a thorough understanding of the subject matter, but also investment of time in terms of obtaining practice in writing' (1984: 75). If you know that each question must be answered in forty minutes, for example, then that is what you must practise, not just once but often. Students who know a topic very well sometimes perform poorly in examinations because they have not learned to select material and write it down in a limited space of time. Some colleges provide students with the opportunity to sit mock examinations, but if yours does not, you can usefully set them for yourself, individually or with a few other students. This will be extremely valuable even if no feedback from the tutor is available. It is also important, in the earlier stages of revision, to practise examination questions in your own time in order to assimilate fully the necessary knowledge. As McIlroy states: 'performing well in examinations is an acquired skill' (1990: 166).

With sufficient examination practice, you should become proficient at completing the entire paper. It cannot be emphasized too strongly how important this is; however successful your answers to three of the questions may be, it is very difficult to do well, or even to pass, if the fourth remains unanswered (Dunleavy, 1986).

It is relatively easy to score the first 20 or 30 per cent of the marks on a question but much more difficult to achieve the later marks; this is illustrated in Figure 4.5.

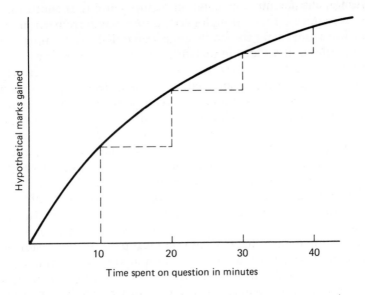

Figure 4.5 *The diminishing returns on time spent per question. (Adapted from Dunleavy P. (1986)* Studying for a Degree in the Humanities and Social Sciences, Macmillan, London, p. 161)

If time is running out and a question has yet to be started, it is essential that you abandon the question you are answering and attempt the final one, even if the only possibility is to sketch a very basic answer plan. If you can only answer three of the four questions, however, it is vital that you keep calm and perform at your optimum with the hope that you may 'scrape through'. In this situation it is often the case that once one or two questions have been answered, confidence is gained, and the fourth, which at first seemed quite impossible, no longer looks so bad.

Probably the most common mistake when taking examinations is failure to answer the questions which are posed. To avoid this it is helpful to underline or highlight key content and instruction words and to refer back to the question frequently. The planning of examination answers is crucial to success; the questions to be answered should be selected with care and a plan made of each before attempting a response. Adequate time must be spent on each part of the question to ensure a well-balanced outcome. On some examination papers the number of marks allocated to each section of the question is indicated; this information is very helpful and careful note should be made of it. Rowntree (1988) believes that it takes nerve, under examination conditions, to spend time thinking and planning, but it is usually time well spent.

An examination paper is no place for repetitive writing. You can only gain the allocated marks *once* for a particular point, so it is useless to make the point again or to exemplify it excessively. It is important that you reach the crux of the issue quickly, the inclusion of irrelevant material wastes time and can obscure the more pertinent points you have made. As with the essay, the examiner will be looking for evidence that you have read round the topic and that you can present your ideas in a reasoned and well-balanced fashion. Fundamental points should not, however, be omitted because they seem too basic or obvious, the examiner should not be left to guess the extent of your knowledge.

Ideally you should leave yourself enough time to read through your answers before leaving the examination room. This will give you the opportunity to insert additional pieces of information, to correct factual errors and grammatical mistakes and to make sure everything is clear. Though tempting, it is usually inadvisable to leave the examination room early.

Although the format of the examination answer and that of the essay will be similar in some respects, the tasks are very different. Students often feel that their written answers in an examination are inadequate, especially later at the coffee and post-mortem stage, or when they read the beautiful essays they previously prepared on the topic. These essay tasks were set, however, so that students could produce a piece of writing over time and with many resources. It is important to remember that the same response is not expected under examination conditions. (For detailed advice on planning and writing assignments, the reader is referred to chapter 2.)

Writing in the clinical setting

When therapy students are in a practical setting, in a hospital, health centre or school, then various other written tasks will be required of them. Records will almost certainly be kept of the treatment given to patients and clients, with different institutions having varying systems for gathering this information. Students need to become acquainted with the system adopted by any particular department and to take advice on precisely how it is used. The rule that writing should communicate is particularly important here; if the treatment given by one therapist is not clearly recorded then it is possible that costly, painful or even dangerous mistakes may subsequently occur.

Some recording systems used in therapy departments have sections which are 'written' only in the sense that a pen is used. In these busy days, writing words is time consuming and you may find yourself confronted by a mixture of symbols, charts, scales, abbreviations and 'tick lists'. Systems rarely rely entirely on symbols such as these, however, for while they may save time, they also select and shape information in ways which may be detrimental to patients. There may, for instance, be no room among the charts and scales for an important and complex perspective from the patient to be recorded (French, 1992).

At the end of a clinical placement, you will almost certainly have the opportunity to read written appraisals about yourself and perhaps to appraise your own performance. Such self-assessment is often thought to be 'worthwhile educationally [as it] encourages openness and honesty about assessment' (Newble and Cannon, 1990: 123).

You may also be asked to write down your views on the clinical placement in general. It is very helpful to plan for this so that nothing worth recording is forgotten. If you receive a disappointing appraisal, you might be tempted to write facetiously or unduly critically of the people whose job it was to help you. When putting your thoughts and feelings into writing, however, it is wise to remain as objective and detached as possible as such documents will remain on file. This having been said, it is important that the opinions of students are acknowledged, valued and acted upon. (For further discussion of writing in the clinical setting, the reader is referred to chapter 5.)

Conclusion

The written tasks demanded of you as a student are very varied and can be difficult to fulfil. Most of the writing you will produce is seen, appraised and marked by others who have had the opportunity to become more knowledgeable, on the particular subject in question, than yourself. This constant scrutiny can be deflating, but should be accepted gratefully, for students, like all writers, need feedback and criticism in order to improve. It is unlikely that such detailed advice will be available to you at any other stage, and you should be encouraged by the thought that it is practically impossible to complete a course of study without emerging a better writer.

5

Clinical Writing

Writing in the clinical field differs from a number of the forms of writing considered elsewhere in this book simply because it is not generally destined for publication. Instead of being made available in the public domain, clinical documents are usually for the use of a fairly circumscribed group of professionals, often based in the same hospital or institution. Notwithstanding this, an equal amount of care must go into clinical writing as into books or articles. Correct use of terminology, avoidance of ambiguity, and general clarity are important features of written communication in all areas of the therapist's professional life. Indeed, it could be argued that these factors are at a special premium in clinical practice, as the safety and well-being of patients and clients may in some cases hinge directly on the quality of the written communication between health professionals.

This chapter will explore three main areas of clinical writing: clinical notes, clinical reports, and writing aimed at patients. As these exemplify between them a range of appropriate styles and approaches, particular attention will be paid to grammatical considerations, and the use of English in general.

Clinical notes

It is self-evident that the clinical care of patients, and their subsequent progress, should be recorded in writing, or in some other permanent medium. Not only is this vital as a means of sharing information with other professionals involved in the treatment programme, it also has important medicolegal implications (see chapter 10).

The form that clinical notes take is therefore extremely important; but so is the way in which they are created. Whatever system you employ, your notes should as far as possible be made at the time, rather than retrospectively. This helps to eliminate the failures of memory to which everybody is prone, especially those in a busy clinical environment. It also facilitates verbatim transcription of statements or dialogues when this is desirable, such as in the assessment of language disorders or speech deficits, or when managing patients with psychiatric problems. However, the need to formulate a comprehensive account of the clinical encounter should not be allowed to undermine the quality of patient–therapist interaction. The therapist whose head is buried in a sheaf of case notes, assiduously copying down every word that is uttered, is likely to detract from, not improve, the overall communication process. Although verbal cues may be documented in minute detail in this way, non-verbal cues are likely to be missed. Moreover, the act of writing tends to involve lack of eye contact and a closed rather than an open posture, which is not conducive to effective two-way communication (Sim, 1993). Consequently, it is often appropriate to wait until a suitable juncture before recording assessment findings, and it may be advisable to leave some aspects of the interaction to be written up once you and the patient or client have parted company.

Another principle to follow is that of making clinical notes as economical as possible. This allows you to create them more efficiently, thereby maximizing the time that is spent in more meaningful interaction with the patient, and it also permits others to familiarize themselves with the content of your notes without having to plough through line upon line of redundant script. Short, familiar words which are easy to spell should be the first choice. In addition, it is quite acceptable to adopt an elliptical writing style, whereby various non-essential pronouns and other words are omitted (e.g. 'Patient has pain in neck since car accident – no direct trauma as far as can recall', 'x-ray seen; irregular lesion right mid-zone').

The use of abbreviations or symbols can also be helpful here, though these can easily be misused. Some abbreviations are well known both within and between professions. Whether you are a physiotherapist, occupational therapist or speech and language therapist, you will almost certainly recognize 'CVA' as an abbreviation for 'cerebrovascular accident', 'CHD' for 'coronary heart disease' or 'DRO' for 'disablement resettlement officer'. However, it may only be speech and language therapists who will read 'NEMD' as 'non-specific esophageal motility disorder' or 'DAD' as 'developmental articulatory dyspraxia', and only those therapists involved in psychiatric care will necessarily take 'FCT' to stand for 'family crisis therapy'. No doubt the vast majority of therapists with any experience of neurological rehabilitation will instantly recognize 'NDT' as 'neurodevelopmental therapy', but few medical practitioners will probably do so. You should also be aware that some abbreviations fulfil more than one use ('PID' is often used to denote both 'pelvic inflammatory disease' and 'prolapsed intervertebral disc') and others are subject to change – 'ADL' ('activities of daily living') is largely being superseded by abbreviations such as 'ILS' ('independent living skills').

Much the same applies to the use of symbols. A symbol like '>' is generally acknowledged to mean 'more than', just as '"' denotes 'inches' – even to those who have long since adopted SI units! The use of '#' to indicate 'fracture' is fairly common practice among workers in orthopaedics. Other symbols may be specific to a particular profession. Manipulative physiotherapists, for example, have a complex array of symbols to describe their techniques. As it is only other physiotherapists familiar with their use who are likely to have to interpret them, there is little scope for misunderstanding. The use of obscure symbols in multidisciplinary case notes, on the other hand, is a likely source of confusion.

Enough has been said to demonstrate that abbreviations and symbols must be used judiciously, with due regard to those who are likely to have to unravel them. It follows that idiosyncratic personal abbreviations – 'GMEAHT' for 'general mobility exercises, advice and home treatment', or 'MOMTTD' for 'maybe one more treatment, then discharge' – should be strictly avoided. For further discussion of the use of abbreviations and symbols, see Kolin and Kolin (1980).

The form of clinical notes

A choice must be made as to which system of clinical notes to use. Notes can be written in the narrative method, in which 'all entries are made in chronological sequence with descriptive details simply relating the events of an incident, treatment, or occurrence without including any type of written conclusion about the given information' (Kolin and Kolin, 1980: 85). However, a more structured approach is generally favoured nowadays.

The Problem Oriented Medical Record (POMR), a system originally developed by Weed (1969), has gained considerable popularity. Briefly, this is a means of recording clinical information in four sections: 'database', 'problem list', 'initial plan' and 'progress notes'. These progress notes are in turn constituted under four headings: 'subjective', 'objective', 'assessment' and 'plan' (these together form the acronym 'SOAP'). Further details of the system and how to operate it can be found in Weed (1969) and Petrie and McIntyre (1979).

There are a number of merits in POMR. There is much to be said for the move from diagnosis-led to problem-led practice, and this is clearly facilitated by POMR. Similarly, the use of a sequential, categorized formula may encourage a thorough and systematic approach to assessment. The POMR system has also shown itself to be capable of use by therapists, nurses and medical practitioners. Advocates of the system further point to the ease with which POMR notes can be computerized, and stress their usefulness in clinical audit.

Against these should be set some significant drawbacks. Some of the technical advantages claimed for POMR, in terms of speed, efficiency and accuracy, have been seriously questioned (Fletcher, 1974). More significantly, the division between 'objective' and 'subjective' which is at the heart of the system may encourage misconceptions (French, 1991). There is a danger that the therapist's findings may be given undue priority over the patient's own views. 'Objective' clinical tests and measurements are not necessarily free from subjective influences, and what the patient has to say about his or her 'subjective' symptoms may be based on highly objective evidence. Objectivity and subjectivity are troublesome concepts, and the POMR system may suggest that they are far more straightforward than is in fact the case. A further criticism is that the system may encourage therapists to believe that patients' problems may be solved by health professionals at a purely individual level, whereas social, economic and political factors may also have to be addressed (French, 1991).

Perhaps in view of criticisms such as these, many practitioners have abandoned the pure POMR format and adopted a modified system. Indeed, Scholey (1985) suggests that such modification is vital in order for the POMR system to be responsive to local and specialized needs. By way of an example, the original POMR system requires that, after a statement of proposed treatment in the initial plan, only subsequent changes in treatment are recorded in the progress notes. If there is no such change, no entry is made. Many therapists are unhappy with the idea that no explicit record is made of the treatment given on each occasion (not least for medicolegal reasons), and modify the system accordingly.

Other clinical tools prescribe not only the general form of the assessment, but also the specific items to be addressed. Such scales or indexes are particularly common in psychiatric and neurological practice; e.g. the Motor Club Stroke Assessment (Ashburn, 1982), the Comprehensive Occupational Therapy Evaluation (COTE) Scale (Hemphill, 1982), and the Clifton Assessment Procedures for the Elderly (CAPE). In many instances, a number of test items have to be scored, in a given order, on a purpose-designed proforma, and an ultimate numerical score can often be derived. These tools have the advantage that individual test items are rarely omitted, as they may be in less formal assessment routines. The tools can also be subjected to systematic testing in terms of validity and reliability, making them suitable for both clinical practice and research. The danger with such instruments, of course, is that instead of the assessment schedule being responsive to the specific clinical features of the patient, the latter is somehow made to fit a preconceived format. The patient's own definition of the problem is particularly prone to being overlooked, or translated into standardized professional terminology. Indeed, some assessment forms, in their search for objective, quantifiable clinical data, make virtually no provision in their design for the patient's perspective. Moreover, unless the targeted group of patients is relatively homogeneous, a given scale or index will rarely be sufficiently flexible to cater adequately for the full range of clinical presentations likely to be encountered – or, if it is indeed flexible enough, it may well lack the necessary degree of specificity. Again, you may feel the need, when using such instruments, to modify, adapt or supplement them. You might, alternatively, wish to combine elements from a variety of standardized instruments into a composite assessment battery; this approach is often helpful when there is a need to construct multidisciplinary assessments.

Adopting a neutral tone

It is important to construct clinical notes without the use of judgemental words or phrases. Your own personal reactions to an individual's personality or physical appearance may be unavoidable, but they should not be recorded in the notes. Not only is this disrespectful to the patient or client concerned, but it is also likely to prejudice the attitudes of other professionals who will subsequently read the notes.

Language which denigrates or stereotypes, such as that discussed in chapter 3, is therefore as undesirable in clinical writing as it is elsewhere. In particular, it is important to avoid adjectives with an evaluative undertone. For example a body part should be referred to as 'flaccid' rather than 'flabby', a gait as 'uncoordinated' rather than 'ungainly', a mood state as 'irritable' rather than 'tetchy' and an abdomen as 'protruding' rather than 'paunchy'. A patient should be recorded as making 'a weak effort', not 'a feeble effort', and relatives should be described as 'anxious' or 'solicitous', not 'fussing' or 'overprotective'.

Clinical reports

Clinical reports may take the form of handwritten entries in the patient's clinical case notes. Alternatively, they may appear as more formally written progress reports or discharge letters, both of which will, in most cases, be subsequently inserted in the case notes. Some points of both good and bad practice will be illustrated by means of an example of a discharge letter.

PHYSIOTHERAPY DEPARTMENT

3rd November 1992

Dr Selsdon
Registrar in Rheumatology
Victoria Building
St Andrew's Hospital
Durham DH4 6RE

Dear Dr Selsdon,

Mrs Joan Forbes

Thank you for referring this lady with shoulder pain, who we first saw in the Physiotherapy Department three weeks ago. Mrs Forbes presented with pain effecting her sleep and limitation of movement in the shoulder, which has since responded to ice, P.N.F. and cervical traction.

Mrs Forbes has reported symptomatic relief for her Osteoarthrosis. If you are agreeable, I will see her once more and then discontinue her Physiotherapy.

Yours faithfully,

J. L. Machin

Above all, this letter is uninformative. On first reading it, the doctor to whom it is addressed will find it hard to connect it with a specific patient (unless the patient's notes are immediately to hand), given that virtually no personal details are provided other than the patient's name and marital status. Moreover, the information given about the initial assessment is extremely brief; ideally, this information should allow the referring doctor to reconstruct, albeit only in outline, the patient's history. It should certainly make it clear which shoulder was treated! The first paragraph could therefore have been phrased in fuller terms, such as:

> Thank you for referring this 54 year-old lady with longstanding generalized osteoarthrosis, who presented with pain and limitation of movement in the left shoulder, following a fall on the 17th October. Mrs Forbes first attended three weeks ago. On examination, all glenohumeral movements were limited, especially abduction, and the patient reported moderately severe pain at the extremes of movement. On cervical spine screening, lack of left rotation was noted. Other assessment findings were unremarkable.

What of the description given in the original letter of the patient's treatment? It would seem that the main components of the treatment programme are provided. However, a valuable opportunity has been lost to enlighten the rheumatologist as to the rationale for the treatment modalities employed. Therapists frequently complain that members of the medical profession inadequately understand their respective rôles and the specific contribution that they each can make to patient care (and, just as important, the contribution that they *cannot* make). The progress report or discharge letter is often the only chance the therapist gets to 'educate' the referring doctor in such matters. The letter above fails to fulfil this purpose. An abbreviation is used ('PNF' for 'proprioceptive neuromuscular facilitation') which will very likely mean little to most doctors. No explanation is given as to why the cervical spine was treated in a patient with an ostensible shoulder problem (such an explanation is provided in the fuller account of the assessment findings suggested above).

Furthermore, the outcome of treatment is sketchy. In order to know whether to give the patient another appointment to attend the out patients clinic, the doctor would find it helpful to know exactly how much symptomatic relief Mrs Forbes has experienced. And what of any improvement in her limitation of movement?

Note also how the therapist's hands have effectively been tied by the final paragraph of the letter, which suggests that the patient's discharge is conditional on the express agreement of the registrar. If no response is received, can the patient be discharged or not? Indeed, the sentence is probably little more than a rather misguided courtesy, as it is questionable whether the physiotherapist need seek sanction for an action which is squarely within his or her own professional discretion.

Again, a better approach might be:

> We have seen Mrs Forbes on five occasions, during which ice has been applied for pain relief, and active exercise (proprioceptive neuromuscular facilitation) has been employed to overcome muscle spasm and increase joint mobility. The limitation of cervical movement indicated a need for mobilization, which was performed by means of manual traction. Mrs Forbes now has approximately 90 per cent of shoulder movement, with respect to the unaffected side, and feels very little pain, such that she can happily lie on her left side. We anticipate discharging her next week, and will provide her with advice for home treatment.

This does, of course, make for a considerably longer letter, and it may be argued that busy clinicians have insufficient time to write anything but the briefest of correspondence. This is an understandable response, but skimping on clinical reports is a wholly false economy; unless a report fulfils its intended purpose, there is no point in spending even a few minutes on producing it.

The final point to be made about the original letter is that it contains some minor but regrettable technical and stylistic shortcomings. Specifically:

— In the recipient's address at the top of the letter, the doctor's initials or forename should have been provided, rather than just his or her surname (though 'Dear Dr Selsdon' is, of course, correct as the salutation).

— In a similar way, the manner in which the letter was signed should have been more explicit. Was this letter in fact from the treating physiotherapist, or from the departmental clerk? To whom should any reply be addressed – Mr Machin, Ms Machin, Dr Machin? A forename or a title should have been supplied.

— The appropriate phrase when concluding a letter to a named individual is 'Yours sincerely', not 'Yours faithfully' (note that in the United States the corresponding phrase is 'Sincerely yours', or just 'Sincerely').

— The strict meaning of the word 'agreeable' is 'pleasant', or 'pleasing'; its colloquial use to mean 'in agreement', or 'willing' should be avoided.

— The word 'effecting' should be 'affecting', and 'has since responded' should be 'have since responded', on the basis that both pain and limitation of movement have presumably been favourably influenced by the modalities stated. Likewise, 'who we first saw' should read 'whom we first saw'.

— The names of diseases or syndromes do not take an initial capital letter, unless they are eponyms (e.g. Raynaud's disease, Alzheimer's disease, Lesch-Nyhan syndrome); hence 'Osteoarthrosis' is incorrect. The same applies to the titles of professions, except when used as, or in conjunction with, a proper noun; thus whereas 'Physiotherapy Department' is correct in the first paragraph, 'Physiotherapy', in the second paragraph, is incorrect. Similarly, one would write 'the Superintendent Physiotherapist advised that a more experienced physiotherapist should assess the patient'.

— Both 'I' and 'we' have been used; the letter should be consistently in either the first person singular or the first person plural.

It may be objected that stylistic and grammatical niceties are insignificant matters, and scarcely warrant more than cursory attention. However, quite apart from the blurring of meaning that can result, the way in which you communicate in writing with your professional colleagues may be the only direct way in which you can form an impression on them. Moreover, as was indicated in chapter 1, all sorts of other shortcomings may be inferred on the basis of inadequate writing ability. Thus, the image which others hold of your professional competence is influenced far more than is at first apparent by the nature and quality of your professional writing.

Finally, it should be remembered that clinical reports are a permanent record which may ultimately be read by many individuals. Whatever professional impression you give of yourself will be enduring and widely disseminated. In a similar way, clinical reports may return to haunt you in future years in the event of their being offered as legal evidence. Both of these considerations point to a high degree of care in their construction.

Writing for patients

Broadly speaking, the writing that you may be called on to produce for patients falls under one of three categories:

(1) Writing for specific patients, or groups of patients, under your care.
(2) Writing for the public or groups of patients in general.
(3) Writing for third parties, such as patients' relatives, employers, lawyers etc.

In each case, the nature and purpose of the communication will dictate the form it should take. It is necessary, therefore, to consider briefly these categories of writing, before going on to address some of the considerations of both style and content which bear upon them:

Writing for specific patients

When writing for patients who are under your care, or with whom you are otherwise familiar, you are usually dealing with individuals whose needs you understand well, and whose level of awareness and understanding you will be familiar with. You will, for example, know the past history of a patient for whom you are writing a programme of home exercises or a list of points of advice. You are able to set such writing within the context of what the patient knows or has previously been told, his or her specific clinical needs, and the nature of the clinical relationship that has been established between yourself and the patient. Even if you are writing for a group of such individuals, much the same assumptions can generally be made.

This sort of clinical writing may therefore have a very specific purpose, and while it may deal with certain points in some detail, other points, which are known to be outside the patients' specific needs, may not be addressed. Anything which is written can be supplemented by oral instructions, and of course vice versa.

Writing for patients in general

This is a different matter. Your readership is not usually identified in any detail. The writing you are producing may be for the general public, in the form of a health education pamphlet; here, you are potentially addressing the whole population. Alternatively, it might be for national charities or self-help groups, such as the National Ankylosing Spondylitis Society or the Multiple Sclerosis Society. In this case, you will have a much fuller understanding of your readership, but this will nonetheless tend to be based on certain general assumptions rather than on a first hand acquaintance with those for whom you are writing.

Writing in this situation, must necessarily be less focused and will have to cater for a far wider spectrum of existing knowledge and understanding. Additionally, there is usually no opportunity to augment the written word with oral explanations.

Writing for third parties

This sort of writing may be directed at patients' relatives who have a high degree of awareness of the matters concerned. On the other hand, it may be intended for employers, teachers or local government officials with a scanty understanding of the issues affecting the patient(s) in question.

Terminology

It is a commonplace of professional practice that technical terminology should be avoided when communicating with patients. We saw in chapter 1 that instructions for patients tend to achieve greater clarity when this principle is observed. However, like all rules of thumb, it requires some qualification. Although an information sheet couched entirely in professional or clinical jargon will in most cases be impenetrable to the majority of patients, this is not a reason for avoiding such vocabulary and phrasing everything in purely lay terminology. Firstly, to do so may be to underestimate the degree of understanding which many patients have of their condition and of medical terms and concepts in general. The public are exposed to a large amount of health-related information in the media, whether in magazines, newspapers or television documentaries, and it is easy to underestimate their knowledge of such matters. Secondly, part of the purpose of information sheets and similar material is to educate patients, and an introduction to some of the technical terms related to their condition would seem to be a necessary part of this process. If you feel that patients will encounter these terms in other contexts, it seems more sensible to provide accurate explanations while you have the chance, than simply to avoid them.

Technical vocabulary need not be totally shunned, therefore, but when it is employed each term should be used with due care as to its likely familiarity to the target readership. In most cases, some sort of definition will be called for. When writing for the general public, a relatively brief explanation may be all that is required:

> When lifting, if you keep your spine flexed (i.e. bent forwards) this will place a strain on the discs, which are the shock-absorbing pads between the bones making up your spine. Instead, you should keep your back as straight as possible.

Similar advice to patients with a specific history of back injury may be more detailed, given that their initial knowledge is likely to be greater, and also that they may require detailed understanding of the underlying mechanisms:

> When lifting, if you keep your spine flexed (i.e. bent forwards) this will place a strain on the intervertebral discs. These shock-absorbing pads between your vertebrae consist of a soft nucleus enclosed in a ring of more rigid tissue, and flexion of the spine can cause the nucleus to bulge at the back of the disc, putting pressure on your nerve roots. Therefore, you should keep your back as straight as possible when lifting.

When writing to third parties, a wide variety of terminology may be appropriate in different cases. Writing aimed at well-informed relatives of patients will essentially follow the principles outlined above. At times, however, you may have to communicate with individuals whose technical knowledge is at a low level, but with whom for various reasons you will have to use specialist language. If you are called upon to write a report on a patient for a solicitor or an insurance company, it may be crucial to give a precise technical account of the patient's condition and the specific treatment administered; to do otherwise could give rise to undesirable legal complications. However, as was suggested earlier, if terms are appropriately defined, specialist vocabulary can be used in such cases without undue bafflement or mystification. Moreover, unlike most patients' relatives, law firms, insurers and most moderately-sized companies generally have ready access to qualified advisors on such matters.

Clarity

An example was given in chapter 1 of writing that could confuse or mislead patients. It is easy to understand how this comes about. The therapist, familiar with his or her intended meaning, may easily write with insufficient awareness of how different, and even contradictory, messages can be drawn by the lay reader. This may be due to apparently minor features of grammar and vocabulary. Consider, for example, this adaptation of the passage quoted above:

> When lifting heavy loads, it is important not to flex your spine (i.e. bend it forwards) as this will place a strain on the spinal ligaments and intervertebral discs. These shock-absorbing pads, located between your vertebrae, consist of a soft nucleus enclosed in a ring of more rigid tissue, and such a movement of the spine can cause the nucleus to protrude at the back of the disc, putting pressure on your nerve roots. Therefore, you should keep your back as straight as possible when lifting. Another thing you should not do to avoid back strain is to sit continually in one position; rather, you should change your sitting posture regularly.

The first thing to strike one here is the suggestion that this advice applies only when lifting *heavy* loads, whereas it is of course important in all acts of lifting. Its importance is, to be sure, heightened when lifting heavy objects, but in trying to emphasize this the writer has unintentionally implied that light lifting tasks are excluded from these recommendations. Note also the ambiguity in the explanation given of spinal flexion. The words 'bend it forwards' are intended to clarify 'to flex your spine', but they could equally be taken to refer to the more complete phrase 'not to flex your spine', and thus convey the opposite meaning. In the following sentence, it is not clear to the lay reader whether the description of the 'shock-absorbing pads' relates only to the intervertebral discs mentioned in the previous sentence, or to both the discs and the spinal ligaments. The professional will not of course make this mistake, but the lay reader may be in genuine confusion here. He or she may also be unsure of the meaning of 'protrude', and a more common word, such as 'bulge' in the earlier extract, should be chosen. The confusion as to movements, which originally surfaced in the first sentence, is now increased, as it is not unmistakably clear which movement is referred to as 'such a movement of the spine'. It might also be suggested that this sentence is longer than it need be, with too many subordinate clauses.

The final sentence could also be improved. In the first place, to refer to an activity as a 'thing you should not do to avoid back strain' is an awkward turn of phrase; indeed, it seems almost to suggest that, although lifting with feet together should not be done to avoid back strain, it is a legitimate activity for certain other purposes! Secondly, by misusing 'continually' (meaning repeatedly) in place of 'continuously' (meaning without break), the writer has given an extremely confusing recommendation. Similarly, one suspects that the writer has followed a common misconception in using the word 'regularly' as a synonym for 'frequently'.

To give written material to patients which is ambiguous is not just ineffective, it may also have serious legal consequences. If advice given to a patient is unclear to the point of being dangerous, it could give rise to a charge of negligence.

Tone

In addition to ensuring that writing for patients and relatives is clear and appropriate in its content, it is important to strike the correct tone. For example it is important to explain facts or procedures in a detailed, methodical manner, but without appearing to patronize. The impression should be given that a detailed explanation is provided for the sake of thoroughness, not because the individual's knowledge or comprehension is thought to be inadequate. The inclusion of a few phrases like 'as you will be aware' or 'it is worth stressing again that' may be all that is required to convey the right tone.

In an attempt to transmit the importance of a piece of advice, it is easy to appear unduly dogmatic or alarmist. The correct balance can be hard to achieve. If you tell patients to 'try to avoid' doing something, they may feel that the injunction is probably unimportant and effectively ignore it, or may have difficulty in distinguishing those occasions when avoidance is important from those on which it is a trivial matter. Alternatively, if you instruct them 'never' to do something, they may take you at your word in a way you never intended. Moreover, if you phrase all your recommendations in peremptory, categorical terms, you will have left yourself with little additional emphasis for those points that are of special importance. Save the strong imperatives for when they are really needed.

Similarly, if you suggest that performing, or failing to perform, a certain activity will produce serious consequences, this may serve as a useful reminder, but it may also cause undue anxiety and lead patients to be unnecessarily cautious. If you paint too dismal a picture in order to reinforce your meaning, the opposite effect may occur, as patients will tend to repress the message. Furthermore, if the dire outcome you mentioned were to come about through another means quite unrelated to their own behaviour, patients might nonetheless attribute its happening to their own action or inaction, with consequent feelings of failure and guilt.

Some practical points

The following list, much of which is derived from Ley (1988), provides a few practical suggestions as to how to improve the readability and comprehensibility of written material for patients.

— Make the appearance and layout of the material as attractive as possible.
— When you have the choice, use short words that are likely to be familiar to the reader (though see our earlier comments on terminology).
— Use short sentences where possible, but introduce some variety in the length of your sentences.
— Locate new items of information at the end of sentences.
— Place the most important information at the beginning and/or end of the material (recall of material so placed tends to be greatest; the so-called primacy and recency effects).
— Use numbering or bulleting to present a series of items (the present list illustrates bulleting).
— Express advice and instructions in concrete terms or in both abstract and concrete terms, rather than in abstract terms alone.
— Use metaphors and analogies sparingly; they can obscure your meaning as easily as enhance it.
— Use appropriate illustrations, both to make your material more attractive and to clarify its meaning.

Conclusion

This chapter has examined three main areas of clinical writing in which the therapist is likely to be involved. Some of the relevant considerations, in terms of both style and content, have been highlighted. Clarity is a vital factor in all areas of professional writing, but it is at a special premium when communicating with or about patients and clients; ambiguity can have serious consequences for safe and effective clinical management.

Chapter

6

Making Use of Bibliographic References

As professional literacy has been increasingly appreciated as an important part of the therapist's rôle, there has been a growing awareness of the need to place written material in the context of other published work. This is one of the main considerations which your readers – whether they be your peers, your students or your educators – will have in mind when they come to evaluate your writing. As new theories of professional practice are developed, and as fresh research data accumulate, you will be expected to marshal the contributions that past and contemporary authors have made to a given topic.

Considerable attention has been directed in the professional literature to this aspect of writing. The identification and location of appropriate material have been explored (Roberts, 1986; Bohannon, 1988; Shearer et al., 1992), and some of the difficulties which therapists may encounter in the process have been highlighted (Arnell, 1985). Meanwhile, considerable attention has been paid to the significance of citation patterns (i.e. how often, and in which publications, authors are themselves subsequently cited) as indices of the prestige of both authors and publications (Dean, 1986; Bohannon, 1987; Bohannon and Gibson, 1986).

The present chapter, however, is concerned principally with more practical matters to do with the functions which textual references may serve and the way in which they should be handled when writing a manuscript. As Anderson et al. (1970: 6) have argued, 'research can become a contribution to a field of knowledge only when it is adequately communicated', and, in line with this principle, you should observe the same standards of clarity and precision in the use of references as in all other aspects of professional writing.

Uses and abuses

A basic, but vital, question to ask yourself is 'for what purposes will I make use of references in my writing?' Perhaps the most important purpose of references is to provide support and evidence for statements, ideas or hypotheses which you are putting forward. Readers are made aware that some substantiation exists for your views and, more significantly, are able to evaluate the relevance and validity of such supporting sources for themselves. Similarly, if you are writing an essay or similar piece of coursework, your assessor will wish to see evidence of relevant background reading. In the process, of course, you are giving credit where it is due, and are (at least partially!) protected from the charge of plagiarizing the ideas of others (see chapter 10). However, do not feel obliged to reference each and every statement you make; it is not always necessary to provide support for readily accepted, uncontroversial claims such as 'in contrast to dysphasia, dysarthria is a disorder of speech rather than of language', or 'psychoses are characterized by varying degrees of loss of touch with reality'.

You can also make use of references to direct readers to a source of more detailed exposition, for which space may not be available in your present work. This is especially appropriate when writing research reports, to provide fuller details of standardized research instruments or established statistical operations. You should work on the general principle that a research report should contain sufficient information for another investigator to replicate the study if required (see chapter 7), and any key items that are not presented in the text itself should certainly be accessible by means of references. A similar rôle may be fulfilled in non-research articles. You may wish to deal with the salient points of a particular issue, and then refer your reader to one or two other sources in which a more comprehensive treatment of the subject may be found. In this way, only those aspects germane to your present argument need be explored at any length in the text, and the location of further details is made known to the interested reader. This allows your work to be read, as it were, on two levels, by both the generalist and the specialist reader.

A third general purpose of references is to provide readers with a literature profile of a subject area, often in the form of a review article. Such a paper provides a critical summary and evaluation of the extant literature in a certain field. As the author of such a paper, you will be expected to have searched the literature comprehensively, and all major relevant sources should generally be represented. If you are writing a thesis or a dissertation, considerable importance will be attached by those marking it to the completeness of your literature review – however, you should still retain a vital element of discrimination when selecting sources to include.

A function which a list of references should *not* serve is that of demonstrating to the readership that you have done your 'homework', or of seeking to add a specious academic weight to your text (Kirby, 1981). The quality of your scholarship should emerge from the text itself, not from the bibliography appended to it. Experienced readers are quick to spot those writers who use a body of references to impress – you're sure to trip yourself up sooner or later if you try to use sources with which you are insufficiently familiar: 'Some authors used to take pride in providing a long list of references, but knowledgeable readers are unfavourably impressed by the extravagant citation of material only marginally relevant to what they are reading' (O'Connor and Woodford, 1978: 36). Dixon et al. (1987: 219) remark pithily that a bibliography 'should not include those [works] you ought to have read but haven't' and Shipman (1988: 143) warns against the misuse of references as a 'mobilisation of famous names to place the work on a par with the established'. He suggests that such a practice may be a stratagem whereby the author seeks to forestall criticism.

Which sources to cite

As a general rule, the most up-to-date literature should be cited, because this material will embody the most recent research evidence, and will furthermore often include an appraisal, or even a refutation, of earlier work. However, there is often value in providing the reader with a historical perspective on the development of a particular field of enquiry, and this may involve your referring to a number of early writings. In particular, it may be relevant to direct the reader to early seminal work, even though this may have subsequently been modified to a considerable degree – e.g. the original statement of the gate control theory of pain (Melzack and Wall, 1965).

Clearly, it is also important to choose, where possible, the most relevant and influential citations. While you should obviously conduct your own appraisal of the importance and relevance of each source, it is wise not to overlook those works which have had a notable impact on professional thinking in the area concerned. This will create a 'common ground' with the existing literature, and permit your readers to discern the key points of contact between past and present contributions to any professional debate. Nonetheless, some apparently 'obscure' citations may prove to have particular relevance to the work in hand, and it is useful to bring these to the notice of others. When material from unfamiliar sources is encountered during the preparation of a manuscript, you should attempt to discover something about the status of the publication concerned, and in particular whether it is peer-reviewed. Articles in such journals will have been subjected to a rigorous process of evaluation by independent referees with recognized expertise or experience in the topic area, and while no substitute for the author's own analysis, this does provide some indication of the value and validity of these papers (Lyne, 1989). Do check, however, that you reference the most accessible source of the material concerned. Readers in the United Kingdom will not thank you for referencing a theory to a dissertation lodged in a South American university (perhaps written in Spanish or Portuguese) if they later discover that much the same theory was also written up (in English) in an international journal.

Although references are generally used to support a certain point of view, there is often merit in also citing authors who may have adopted a contrary stance. The more controversial the issue, the more this is appropriate. Not only does this give you the opportunity to weigh up the merits of conflicting perspectives in the text, but the reader too, by following up the relevant citations, can reach his or her own conclusion in much the same way.

How many references should you use? It is certainly not a case of the more the better: 'An absence of references is suspicious, but so is a surfeit. The first possible misuse of references to look out for is over-abundance' (Shipman, 1988: 143). Indeed, some publications (such as the *British Medical Journal*) suggest a maximum number of references for certain categories of article. Even if no such limit is stipulated, when it comes to substantiating a particular point, it is not usually necessary to cite more than two or three sources. Exceptionally, this number may be exceeded; for example, if the very point you want to stress is the unanimity of opinion on an issue, or in the course of a review article, whose purpose is often to evaluate *all* of the germane literature on a subject. However, judicious use of '*inter alia*' ('among others') will often have the desired effect with greater economy.

On occasions, you may find it necessary to access material via secondary sources (i.e. by means of references or quotations in another author's work) if the primary source is particularly difficult to obtain. This is generally an unsatisfactory habit, as it means relying on another writer's interpretation of the original work. Dudley (1977: 23) finds little in the practice to recommend it:

> Better to be guilty of the sin of omission than to adopt the corrupt tendency of making the references for a paper by the appropriation of whole chunks of reference material for quotation from other papers without this being checked or read in the original.

Such use of secondary sources has been shown to lead to inaccurate quotation of original findings and conclusions (De

Lacey et al., 1985). A further consequence is that you may unwittingly reproduce erroneous conclusions, or even falsified data, which have subsequently been retracted. This issue is addressed by Dickersin and Hewitt (1986), who point out that the MEDLINE database produced by the National Library of Medicine now incorporates a subject heading 'Retraction of publication'.

Systems of referencing

There are many different styles of referencing. O'Connor (1978) speaks of a staggering 2632 possible variations, and reports a colleague's finding that a sample of 52 scientific journals shared 33 different styles between them. Mercifully, there is some degree of consensus among publishers and editors, and two systems are predominant; these are the Harvard and the Vancouver styles, or variants thereof. The choice of which system to use is frequently not open to you, as it will have been dictated by the requirements of the publication to which your finished manuscript is to be sent, or by the preferred style of the educational institution you are attending. Nonetheless, it is useful to be aware of the main features of the styles in common use, if only because they will serve as an illustration of some of the broader principles involved in the use of bibliographic references.

The Vancouver style

In this format, references in the text are denoted by consecutive numbers, usually as superscript or in square parentheses. At the end of the text, the works cited are listed in the order in which they appeared. This style is used by *Physical Therapy*, the *British Journal of Occupational Therapy*, *Physiotherapy Canada* and *Clinical Rehabilitation*. It is endorsed by the International Committee of Medical Journal Editors (ICMJE, 1982), which embraces such journals as *Annals of Internal Medicine*, *New England Journal of Medicine* and the *British Medical Journal*.

Generally, in standard Vancouver usage, any given source is referred to throughout by the same number. References to different pages can be given in conjunction with the numeral in the text – e.g. Corbin[46 p126]. However, a variation may be found whereby a fresh number is used each time the source is mentioned. In this case, any page reference will be found not in the textual reference, but in the list. It also means that the citation can be combined with a footnote, as in the following example (which, like all others in this chapter, is fictitious):

34 Dean G.H. Wilcockson R. *Principles of cardiovascular measurement*, New York, Webster and Fulbright, 1987, p 346.
35 Macklovitz J. Cardiac telemetry: a new protocol. *Br J App Cardiol* 1977; 45: 145–148.
36 Dean G.H. Wilcockson R. *op. cit.*, p 450. This method has been used in most of the physiological studies previously reviewed, but has yet to gain acceptance in clinical practice.

This usage is common in theses and other works of a highly scholarly nature, but is rare in journal articles and most books in the therapy professions.

Further variations on the general theme may be found. For example, more than one work may be designated by a given number, and on occasions the references themselves may appear at the foot of the relevant page rather than at the end of the article or chapter. However, both these practices are most common in the humanities and social sciences, and relatively unusual in biomedical journals.

The Harvard style

This is the system used by the *American Journal of Occupational Therapy*, the *Australian Journal of Physiotherapy*, *Physiotherapy*, the *European Journal of Disorders of Communication* and the *British Orthoptic Journal*, and is advocated by the British Standards Institution (BSI, 1976). Authors are identified in the text by name and date in parentheses (or the date alone if the author has already been named in the sentence), and the list of references at the end is in alphabetical order. A variant adopted by *Physiotherapy Theory and Practice*, and used by the publishers Churchill Livingstone as their house style, is the CIBA system; this is the same in all significant aspects, and differs mainly in the minimal use of punctuation and the absence of italics. Generally, the Harvard style has gained greater popularity than the Vancouver system, but in medical journals the opposite trend would seem to be taking place (Lock, 1982). The way in which references are presented in the list differs slightly in the Harvard˙style. For example the references given earlier in Vancouver format would generally appear in a journal using the Harvard style as follows:

> Dean, G.H., & Wilcockson, R. (1987) *Principles of Cardiovascular Measurement*, Webster and Fulbright, New York, p 346.
> Macklovitz, J. (1977) Cardiac telemetry: a new protocol. *British Journal of Applied Cardiology*, 45, 145–148.

In the simplified CIBA system, they would become:

> Dean GH, Wilcockson R 1987 Principles of cardiovascular measurement. Webster and Fulbright, New York, p 346
> Macklovitz J 1977 Cardiac telemetry: a new protocol. British Journal of Applied Cardiology 45: 145–148

The hybrid system

On occasions, you may encounter a format which is essentially a combination of the Harvard and Vancouver styles. The textual references are numbered as in the latter system, but the list of references is given in alphabetical order, rather than in the order of appearance in the text. This style is not often seen in journal articles or chapters in edited volumes, but is more common in books which have a single substantial bibliography at the end.

Pros and cons of the main systems

If you have a choice as to which system to use, you should weigh up their relative merits before deciding in favour of one or the other. There are several advantages to the Harvard system as compared to the Vancouver format. For example the inclusion of the names of the authors in the text often makes it easy for the reader to identify a work when subsequently mentioned without repeatedly turning to the list of references. This is particularly useful when a large number of sources are being compared and contrasted on a number of points. From your point of view as a writer, this same feature makes errors less likely; it is much more probable that the wrong number will be inserted than the wrong name(s). Moreover, the inclusion of new sources in a redraft merely requires you to insert one or more new entries in the reference list, and does not necessitate renumbering all of the subsequent citations, as is the case in the Vancouver system. With this consideration in mind, O'Connor and Woodford (1978) recommend that the preliminary drafts of an article should always use the Harvard style: if a numerical system is required by the publication chosen for submission, it should be substituted in the final draft.

If the nature of your work is such that you sometimes wish to include supplementary material at various points, but without breaking the flow of the text itself, you can accomplish this by the use of footnotes. In the Vancouver system, numerals obviously cannot be used for footnotes unless they are combined with citations (as previously illustrated), and a rather less satisfactory series of symbols is generally resorted to (e.g. *, †, §, **, ††, §§ etc). In the Harvard system, of course, numerals can be used for footnotes, and they are helpfully distinguished in the text from the name-and-date citations. Do note, however, that most journals discourage the use of footnotes; you are more likely to use them in dissertations or theses.

On the other hand, the Harvard style has certain disadvantages. Quoting several sources at a given point in a review article may itself run to a line or more of text, whereas the corresponding Vancouver numerals occupy very little space and do not impede the flow of the text. Also, differentiating several works by the same or similar authors is slightly cumbersome, necessitating as it does careful attention to the listing of names, and the use of letters to distinguish otherwise identical items – e.g. James and Hodgkinson (1987a).

If you are writing a lengthy article with an extensive reference list, the Vancouver format indicates to your readership – by virtue of the consecutive numbering – the approximate place in the text at which a work is first mentioned; this allows the reference list to be used as a sort of index to the article. On the other hand, the Harvard alphabetical listing does permit the reader to ascertain swiftly whether or not a certain author has been cited, even if it gives less indication as to where in your text this has occurred. Furthermore, a number of works by one author will appear together in the Harvard listing (provided of course that he or she is the first-named author in each case), and this may be helpful to the reader in some instances.

As we have pointed out, the choice of target publication usually determines which form of referencing is to be used. Fortunately, most of the work likely to be published in the therapy professions accommodates itself fairly satisfactorily to either of the two principal systems outlined above.

Preparation and presentation

Here, as in all aspects of professional writing, it is important to adopt a systematic approach. Anderson et al. (1970) recommend that a 'working bibliography' should be built up on index cards. Such a system makes it easy to add new sources, and all the items can be readily put into either numerical or alphabetical order, as required by the chosen reference style. You should make a point of recording *all* relevant details, so as to avoid having to search for the relevant volume again in order to discover the author's initials, or to identify the volume number. The reverse of the card can be used for brief notes on the text, and for details such as the library class number. A microcomputer or word processor is a useful alternative to index cards, but is of course far less portable if you are likely to visit a number of libraries or work in more than one place.

References in the text

When presenting citations in the body of the text, you should do so in a way that is informative and unambiguous, for the reader will very likely be unfamiliar with many of the sources that you quote.

The way in which you introduce a reference is significant. When alluding to research findings, it is most appropriate to use such phrases as: 'it has been demonstrated by Brechin et al (1988) that . . .'; 'Brechin et al's (1988) study reveals that . . .'; 'empirical support for this view is to be found in Brechin et al. (1988) . . .', etc. Again mindful of the reader's probable unfamiliarity with the specific material being cited, it is sometimes helpful to give brief additional details of the particular study, such as the size and composition of the sample, whether randomized and/or controlled, whether a pilot or a large multi-centre project, etc.

If, however, you are referring to non-research papers, different phraseology is required; for example 'Robinson (1976) has argued that . . .'; 'it has been proposed by Robinson (1976) that . . .'; 'Robinson's (1976) view is that . . .'. Your readers are immediately alerted to the fact that opinions, propositions and theories are being dealt with, rather than empirical findings.

There will be occasions when you wish to provide examples in the form of citations. As so often, there is a potential danger of ambiguity, which you should guard against. For example in the following sentence – 'Many studies in this area have insufficient validity (Moran, 1979; Johnson, 1985)' – it is not clear whether Moran and Johnson are examples of the deficient studies referred to, or whether they are the proponents of this view. Thus, if you wish to convey the first meaning, greater clarity would be achieved by inserting the citations after the word 'studies' or by adding 'e.g.' before the first citation. If, on the other hand, you intend the second meaning, you could rephrase the sentence to read 'As Moran (1979) and Johnson (1985) have maintained, many studies in this area . . .'.

Similarly, when representing the views of another author, you should make it clear where the quotation or paraphrase ends and your commentary or exposition resumes. Paraphrase can present particular problems. It is difficult, for example, to tell whether the second sentence in the following extract is drawn more or less directly from Pfalzer's argument, or represents the author's own elaboration on this theme:

> Pfalzer (1988) has pointed to the lack of rigour in studies of the management of expressive dysphasia. Few studies have been adequately controlled, samples are all too often insufficiently representative, and research designs have often neglected to utilize an assessor blinded to the treatment allocation.

This problem is unlikely with a direct quotation. Furthermore, if the views expressed in the original are in some measure ambiguous, a direct quotation allows the reader to evaluate the various possible meanings at their source.

Direct quotations from periodical articles can be referenced in the usual way, but those drawn from books should generally indicate the relevant page number so that your readers can verify the quotation without undue effort (do, however, keep a note of the page number(s) of *all* quotations you use, for future reference, and in case you are required by a publication or an educational institution to page-reference every quotation). If only one reference is made to the volume in question, some publications recommend that the page number be included in the reference list; if there is more than one quotation the page number must, of course, follow each of these as they occur in the text. Ensure that you reproduce direct quotations exactly as they appear. Resist the temptation to anglicize American spellings (and vice versa), or to convert alternative spellings to those of a particular publication's house style. Any omission should be designated by an ellipsis (a series of periods), and any explanatory comment you wish to make within the body of the quotation should appear in square parentheses, to make it clear that it is your own interpolation and not part of the original quotation:

> Writing from the perspective of a community service in a rural area, Hussein (1978) points out that 'ever since this system [self-referral in cases of deterioration] has been introduced, client satisfaction has demonstrably increased'.

Similarly, if you are incorporating a quotation into a sentence of your own it may be necessary to change a capital letter in the original to lower case – again, do so by enclosing the changed letter in square parentheses:

> Squires (1991) maintains that '[t]he main obstacle to post-registration education in speech and language therapy is the lack of budgetary control over the appropriate funds'.

Note, however, that according to Hart (1983) a quotation of five lines or more is usually best broken off (i.e. given a paragraph of its own).

If it is desired to emphasize any word or phrase by italicizing it, this should be explained after the citation by the phrase 'emphasis added'; indeed, where the emphasis is present in the original source it may be worth pointing this out also ('emphasis in original'). If the passage chosen contains a misspelt word or an apparent factual error, don't be tempted to correct it. Rather, place the word '*sic*' (Latin for 'thus') in square parentheses immediately following it. Endeavour to resist the temptation of misusing '*sic*' as a means of conveying ironic disagreement with the views expressed by the quoted writer. If you want to take issue with the original author, do so explicitly following the quotation, justifying your bone of contention!

Mistakes in quotations (direct or by means of paraphrase) are all too common. De Lacey et al. (1985) randomly selected fifty quotations from the first issue in 1984 of six medical journals. The overall prevalence of misquotations was 15 per cent, and of these approximately two-fifths were classed as 'seriously misleading'.

Despite our earlier recommendation to avoid them where possible, it may occasionally be necessary to use secondary sources. It is crucial, when you do so, that this is made clear to your readers, to alert them to the fact that you have not had direct access to the original source. This may be achieved thus: 'and a team of Canadian workers (Jacobs et al., 1985, cited in Richards, 1987) have demonstrated that blood pressure remains stable during this manoeuvre.'

If the Vancouver system is being used, the textual reference consists merely of a rather uninformative number. It may therefore be useful to phrase the sentence concerned in such a way as to convey additional information about the provenance and date of the source. For example instead of saying 'vigorous physiotherapy has been shown to be ineffective in this syndrome[14]' the author could say 'Dorlund and Westergen's investigations[14] have shown that vigorous physiotherapy . . .', or 'as long ago as 1971[14] it was demonstrated that vigorous physiotherapy . . .'. In Harvard usage, the date appears alongside the author's name, and should, generally speaking, be repeated each time you cite the source in question. However, provided that no possible ambiguity exists as to exactly which item is being referred to, it is sometimes acceptable to omit the date on a subsequent occasion: 'Rosenberg (1978) and Donaldson and Sumner (1983) have both examined this phenomenon in school-age children. Rosenberg used a same subject design with a sample of girls between the ages of 11 and 14.'

Earlier in this chapter we considered the question of how many sources to cite. Whatever number you decide upon, you will need to consider the order in which they should appear. Essentially you have two choices: alphabetical or chronological order. The latter is rather more meaningful, and is probably the system to be preferred. However, when listing items in date order you should heed two pieces of advice given by Harris (1986). Firstly, do not separate works by the same author by other workers' references that intervene chronologically; list all items by a given writer at the point determined by his or her earliest work. Secondly, use alphabetical listing for items by different authors that appeared in the same year.

Finally, you may sometimes wish to refer to unpublished material. This may involve manuscripts that are in the process of publication, but are yet to appear. O'Connor and Woodford (1978: 54) give the following advice:

> If you cite a paper that has been submitted for publication, do not include it in the reference list unless you are sure that you will be able to change 'submitted for publication' to 'in press'

plus the name of the journal by the time your own paper is likely to be in proof.

It is worth noting that some journals, such as the *Journal of Advanced Nursing*, do not accept references that are listed as 'accepted for publication'.

Alternatively, you may want to refer to materials that are not intended for publication. These are normally designated in the text by such phrases as 'unpublished data' or 'personal communication'. It is generally felt that such references should *not* also appear in the reference list at the end of the manuscript; in this way readers are reminded 'that the work has not been exposed to the critical appraisal of editors and referees, and that it is not readily available for critical study' (O'Connor and Woodford, 1978: 54). This does not apply to theses and dissertations, which, although unpublished work, should normally be listed in the usual way. Conference proceedings are also listed normally, with particular care that all relevant details for their location are included. Bear in mind that there are also ethical considerations involved in citing unpublished material (see chapter 10).

The list of references

It is vital that you give all details of the work concerned in full. By this stage in your writing, you will probably have undergone the frustrating experience of trying to track down an inaccurately referenced source – don't put your readers through the same ordeal! In any case, sloppy referencing detracts unnecessarily from an otherwise accomplished book or article. Furthermore, a needlessly unfavourable impression is created in editors and referees, and this may even tip the balance against acceptance of your work. By the same token, if you are writing a piece of coursework, you may lose marks. It would appear from Poyer's (1979) findings that inaccurate citations are all too common; he found that, in 102 articles examined from 34 journals, 367 of the 2496 references (i.e. approximately 15 per cent) contained at least one error, and that only five bibliographies were free of mistakes. In the study referred to previously, De Lacey et al. (1985) noted that the overall prevalence of erroneous citations was 24 per cent, of which about a third were deemed to be 'major' (i.e. they prevented immediate identification of the source of the reference).

Among the more common errors to guard against are: omitting the town of publication of a book, inaccurate pagination or confusing volume number and part number in a journal article, failing to list all authors of a publication, neglecting to indicate the editor of an edited volume, omitting to specify the edition of a book if other than the first, spelling an author's name differently in text and list, failing to ensure that all textual references are represented in the list (and vice versa), and ignoring the alphabet when placing items in order.

Some journals insist that journal titles be abbreviated according to a specified system (ANSI, 1969). You must, of course, follow the journal's requirements. However, where you have the choice, we would recommend that you give titles in full, as abbreviation has certain drawbacks. In the first instance, whereas some abbreviated titles are well known or easy to interpret (e.g. Am J Occup Ther, Rheumatol Rehabil), others are less so (e.g. Regul Pept, Dig Dis Sci). In addition, the resulting entry is often awkward to read, and the possibility of error and misunderstanding is increased. On the other hand, lengthy bibliographies can be significantly shortened by such abbreviations, and their use is perhaps justified in such cases.

Ensure there is no possible ambiguity in matching textual references with those in the list. For example suppose you intended to cite two papers published in 1987, one by Peters H. A., Rogerson N. and Brien G. T., and one by Peters H. A., Rogerson N., Brien G. T. and Wishart V. In the list of references these would be readily distinguished. However, confusion would occur if they were both referred to as 'Peters et al., 1987' in the text. Thus, despite the fact that the full references differ and would be readily distinguished in their full form, they should be differentiated, in both the text and the list, by the use of '1987a' and '1987b', as described earlier.

If you are using a numerical system, there is the option, as noted above, of using a fresh number for each occasion on which a given source is referenced. In such a case, there are a number of space-saving conventions which you can use. Instead of repeating the full reference on subsequent occasions, *op. cit.* (short for *opere citato*, 'in the work cited') can be used. Alternatively, if the item referenced is the same as the immediately preceding item, *ibid.* (*ibidem*, 'in the same place') can be used. Finally, if you wish to refer to the same page in a previously referenced work, *loc. cit.* (*loco citato*, 'in the passage cited') can be employed to designate this. These can be illustrated by adapting the previous example:

34 Dean G. H., Wilcockson R. *Principles of cardiovascular measurement*, New York, Webster and Fulbright, 1987, p 346.
35 Macklovitz J. Cardiac telemetry: a new protocol. *Br J App Cardiol* 1977; 45: 145–148.
36 Khan J. *Essentials of cardiology*, Seattle, Clinical Science Press, 1983, p 244.
37 Dean G. H., Wilcockson R. *op. cit.*, p 450. This method has been used in most of the physiological studies previously reviewed, but has yet to gain acceptance in clinical practice.
38 *Ibid.*, p 455.
39 Khan J. *loc. cit.*
40 Khan J. *op. cit.*, p 248.

Although the economy that results is apparent, so too is the potential for error. In particular, the insertion of new items not only requires you to renumber subsequent references, but may also necessitate other changes. Thus, a fresh reference between 37 and 38 would mean that 38 (which would become 39, of course) would have to be changed from '*Ibid.*' to 'Dean G. H., Wilcockson R. *op. cit.*, p 455'. The safest course is only to insert these abbreviations in the final draft, when all other changes have been made. Incidentally, do not be tempted to use *ibid.* or *op cit.* in textual references in the Harvard format. Apart from the fact that it is not normal practice, to do so will distract and disconcert your readers, as they are obliged repeatedly to look back in the text to locate the 'parent' reference.

Finally, there may be works which you are eager to draw to the attention of readers but which you have not cited in the text. Following the distinction advocated by Young (1987), these should not be listed among the textual references, but in a separate list headed 'Bibliography'. Cormack (1984) draws attention to the possible use of an 'annotated bibliography', in which each item is accompanied by a short notice or commentary. He points out that such a bibliography is especially valuable in student coursework.

Conclusion

The judicious and appropriate use of citations is an important element in professional writing. Although you will generally be obliged to follow the referencing requirements of individual publications, a familiarity with the various alternatives and their pros and cons will help to give you an insight into the full potential of referencing, and to avoid some of the pitfalls associated with their use.

Chapter

7

Writing a Research Report

Research is becoming an increasingly important part of the therapist's professional rôle. The need to justify professional activity in terms of its demonstrated effectiveness has always been paramount, but it has gained a fresh urgency, in the United Kingdom at least, with rapid reorganization and rationalization of the health services. It hardly needs to be said that carrying out a piece of research is of little value if its results are not made known to the professional community. Although research findings can usefully be disseminated through a number of media, the written word is perhaps the most important of these. Nonetheless, it is common to find researchers who regard the writing up and dissemination of their findings as a tedious and uninteresting task, to be carried out after the 'real' work has been completed. In truth, the process of writing up is at least as important as any other part of the research process. Moreover, it is usually the only basis on which others can evaluate your research, and your reputation will tend to stand or fall by your reports. Similarly, in the case of a student research project, the overwhelming burden of assessment usually falls on the written report.

The research report is thus becoming an important component of professional writing for therapists, and is a form of writing which, above all others perhaps, requires particular care if it is to fulfil its aims and objectives successfully.

General considerations

The basic purpose of writing a research report is to communicate research findings concisely and unambiguously to your intended readership. In line with this general aim, there are a number of rules and principles which are worth observing in the process of writing a scientific paper. However, any guidelines followed should not be regarded as hard and fast, as these will need modification and adaptation in the light of three general considerations, namely:

The type of research report

Generally speaking, there are three principal forms of research report which you may be called upon to write. Firstly, there is a dissertation, thesis or similar report forming part of the assessment on an educational programme. Here, you are not only presenting your findings, you are also displaying, in detail, the way in which they were arrived at. The process of the research is presented for scrutiny (and assessment) as well as its outcome. Secondly, you may choose to write your report for publication in a professional journal. This is the medium through which you communicate your research findings to your professional peers. A report such as this will go through a process of peer review to ensure that it meets the necessary standard for inclusion in the corpus of professional literature (Lyne, 1989; for a discussion of problems to do with peer review see Smith, 1988). Again, the process of the research should be adequately described so that the validity of your findings can be evaluated. In comparison to a dissertation, space is very limited in a journal article – indeed, some journals specify word limits for submissions – and it is important to express yourself as concisely as possible. Finally, there is what could be called an 'informal' research report. You may well wish to present an account of your research in a non-peer-reviewed publication, such as a magazine, newspaper, or professional magazine such as *Therapy Weekly*. The accent here is predominantly on presenting and discussing your findings, and there is not so great a need as in previous cases to give an account of the research process itself.

Style of research

You will find that different methodological approaches to research dictate certain variations of emphasis in your report. The way in which you would construct a report of an experimental, quantitative study will differ from how you would write up a piece of non-experimental, qualitative research. An attempt will be made to highlight these differences when we come to discuss the details of report writing.

The intended readership

This will, of course, be determined largely by the type of report you write, as discussed above – or perhaps it is more accurate to say that your target readership will determine the sort of report you write. Theses and dissertations are classified as 'unpublished' work, and they may only be read by those assessing them within an educational establishment, and perhaps by others doing similar research at a comparable level. In the case of a journal paper, however, your report passes into the public realm and will be exposed to the profession at large. Depending on the journal to which you choose to submit, you may reach either a general or a specialist professional readership. Your work may also, of course, come to the notice of members of other professions. Although 'informal' research reports may be targeted at a specialist branch of the profession, in many cases your potential readership is extremely wide, and may include the general public. Note also that it is quite common to publish research findings in the form of both a journal paper and a magazine article, though the style and approach of the piece would differ significantly in each case.

Structure and content of the research report

With these preliminary comments in mind, we will now examine in some detail the structure and content of a research report. It is customary to do so under headings relating to the various sections of an experimental research report – i.e. title and abstract, introduction, methods, results, discussion, conclusion. We will follow this convention, but with the caveat that these headings may not be appropriate in all cases. In other words, the pattern we will be following should not be taken as the 'gold standard' for all research reports. The relevant changes in emphasis will be highlighted.

Title and abstract

The title chosen should be concise yet informative. At the same time, because it is almost certainly the first part of your report that will be seen, it should stimulate the curiosity of the reader to read further. Make it clear that your paper is a research report. A title such as 'Sensory integrative therapy in brain-injured children' is fairly ambiguous in this regard, whereas 'A controlled trial of sensory integrative therapy in brain-injured children', or 'Sensory integrative therapy in brain-injured children: an empirical study', make it clear that the article to follow will describe a piece of research. Sometimes, researchers choose a title that conveys their main finding, e.g. 'Counselling hastens rehabilitation of below-knee amputees'; however, this may give a rather dogmatic impression of the conclusions you have reached! Remember that colleagues who are searching the literature through indexes without abstracts, such as *Index Medicus* or *Occupational Therapy Index*, will have little other than the title to go on when deciding whether to pursue a given item. You can save them a lot of wasted effort if you make sure that you choose a title which is informative.

When submitting a paper to a journal, the title page will also carry various other details, such as the names of the author(s) and the address for communication. It is usual to list authors in descending order of the contribution that they made to the research itself. Thus the principal researcher would generally appear first. However, only those who were directly involved in the project should be listed; those individuals who gave specialist advice or other forms of support should be acknowledged at the end of the report (see below). If all authors made an approximately equal contribution to the work, alphabetical listing is the convention (though if a project spawns a number of papers, researchers sometimes take it in turns to be first-named author). It is generally assumed that all authors share responsibility for all parts of the report. Consequently, you should avoid what Day (1989: 22) terms the 'laundry list' approach, which involves 'naming as an author practically everyone in the laboratory, including technicians who may have cleaned the glassware after the experiments were completed'. The institutional affiliation is also given for each author. If you have changed your place of work subsequent to carrying out a piece of research, but prior to reporting it, you should publish under your original position, and give your present affiliation in a footnote or similar format.

The abstract, or summary, serves as a very brief précis of your report. O'Connor and Woodford (1978) describe two sorts of abstract. An 'informative' abstract, which they recommend for research reports, consists of a series of factual statements covering the key elements of the report itself. The essentials of the research question or hypothesis, the research design adopted, the means of data analysis utilized, the data obtained, together with the conclusions drawn from them, should all be available in the informative abstract. An 'indicative' abstract differs somewhat, as it aims to provide not so much a precise summary of the paper as a general guide to its contents, indicating the issues addressed and the general line of argument pursued. Indicative abstracts are more suited to papers such as review articles or those expounding theoretical issues. The key fact to bear in mind when constructing an abstract is that it should be capable of being read independently of the paper to which it refers – indeed, abstracts are commonly reproduced separately. Thus, everything you write in the abstract should be intelligible to the reader without the need for recourse to the text of the paper itself. Cormack's claim that the abstract 'should accurately summarize the *entire* contents of the work' (Cormack, 1984: 102, original emphasis) requires some qualification. As we have noted, all the key elements of the paper should be addressed – but this is not to say that everything in your paper will be represented in the abstract. However, the abstract must not include anything that does not appear in the main text. In view of these considerations, it is wise not to begin writing the abstract until all other sections of the paper have been completed.

Resist the temptation to include technical details that are likely to be unfamiliar to non-specialists and/or are peripheral to the key features of the study. Unless there are pressing reasons for doing so, do not include bibliographic references in the abstract (if they must appear, ensure that they are given in full).

If the manuscript you are preparing is for publication in a journal, you may be required to select between three and five key words, so that your paper can be indexed. The assistance of an experienced librarian can be extremely valuable here.

Introduction

There are a number of issues which you should address in the introduction:

(1) the overall aims of the study;
(2) how the study fits into existing knowledge in the area concerned;
(3) why it was worth carrying out, and particularly its relevance to professional practice;
(4) the type of study undertaken, in terms of its general design and methodological approach;
(5) the research question or hypothesis being examined.

It is probably helpful to address these points in more or less the order in which they are listed above. Harris (1986) recommends that you should move from the general to the specific as you proceed through your introduction. Thus, having given a very brief statement of the general purpose of the study (1), you move into a consideration of the underlying theoretical issues and a critical review of the existing literature relevant to the area concerned (2). This then enables you to justify the need for your particular study, perhaps by pointing to a paucity of previous research on the particular topic which you intend to investigate, or by identifying certain trends in clinical practice which have indicated a gap in professional knowledge (3). Finally, you can consider the specifics of your own study (4 and 5). In particular, you should give a clear statement of your research question or hypothesis. You need not, however, give any great detail as to the design and methods that you adopted – to do so would be to pre-empt material that you will be presenting in the next section of your paper. It is probably sufficient to state that the study took the form of a randomized controlled clinical trial, a within-subjects experimental design, an attitude survey using a questionnaire, a covert participant observation study or whatever.

When reviewing the literature, you may wish to do this as an integral part of your introduction, or you may wish to create a sub-heading specifically for this purpose. What method you opt for will probably be determined by the quantity of relevant literature, and the complexity of the issues which it raises. In the case of a thesis or dissertation, you may even wish to grant the literature review a section of its own, as the review will almost certainly be expected to be considerably more wide-ranging than that presented in a published research report. In all cases, however, it is important to strike the right balance between comprehensiveness and discrimination when selecting those items to discuss. Guidance on how to handle bibliographic sources is given in chapter 6.

In the course of reviewing the literature, you may find that various authors have interpreted certain terms or concepts in slightly different ways. It is important that you establish clearly in your introduction the definition(s) which you intend to follow, and how these relate to those adopted by previous researchers. Do not simply assume that the definition of a concept such as nominal aphasia or neuromuscular fatigue is self-evident. Provide an explicit working definition, and if this is based on earlier work, provide the appropriate reference(s). If some workers have relied on an alternative definition which you regard as unsatisfactory or insufficient, you should address this issue explicitly.

It is important to remember that you do not necessarily have to present a hypothesis as such. A hypothesis is merely a particular sort of research question which is suited to some forms of research. Where you have a fairly specific, closely-focused research question, you may be in a position to state this in the form of the expected results – 'transcutaneous nerve stimulation (TNS) gives superior pain relief to ice therapy in cases of tennis elbow'. This would be your hypothesis, which your study results would cause you either to retain or to reject. On the other hand, the topic you propose to study might not lend itself to a clear-cut prediction of the findings. For example you might wish to examine patients' attitudes to joint goal-setting in speech and language therapy consultations. There would possibly be a number of different strands to this question – whether patients regard joint goal-setting as an important element in their treatment, whether their image of the therapist is affected accordingly, the perceived nature and extent of their own involvement in the process etc. Additionally, there may be no grounds on which to predict the sorts of responses you are likely to obtain on these issues. Consequently, in a case like this, a research question in general terms is called for – perhaps little more than 'What attitudes do patients hold towards the use of joint goal-setting in the context of speech and language therapy?'

If you intend to test your hypothesis by means of inferential statistics, you should also have a null hypothesis (your original hypothesis is known as the experimental or alternative hypothesis). In the example given earlier, the experimental hypothesis would be that manipulation of the independent variable in a certain way (i.e. manipulating the type of treatment given: TNS or ice) would have a specific effect on the dependent variable (i.e. superior pain relief with TNS). The null hypothesis is the contradictory of this. It predicts that there is no such effect, i.e. that the stated difference in pain relief between ice and TNS will not be found (note that it does not posit the opposite effect, namely that ice is superior to TNS). In the course of statistical inference, you will seek to support your experimental hypothesis indirectly, by disproving the null hypotheses – further details on the rationale for this are given in Hicks (1988: 35–39). As the null hypothesis always takes the same form, it is not always necessary to state it in a research report in a periodical; the reader can infer it from your experimental hypothesis. In a thesis or dissertation, however, where we have noted the need to be very explicit about all the procedures followed, you should include the null hypothesis.

The final point to be made about the introduction is that, although the entire report will probably be written after the completion of the study, you should, as far as possible, reflect the temporal sequence of the project as a whole. In other words, the introduction should refer to the preparatory and design stages of the study, and not to aspects, such as the results and the conclusions drawn from them, which have not 'happened' yet.

The introduction to a research report can be seen, at its simplest, as providing an answer to the question 'what did you set out to investigate, and what led you to do so?'

Methods

This section may appear under a variety of names – 'methods', 'subjects and methods', 'methodology', 'materials and methods'. Its purpose, however, is the same – to describe the various procedures that were carried out during the actual conduct of the research, together with a justification for their choice.

It is usual to begin by describing the subjects of the research in terms of such features as their age, sex, occupation, disease status etc. The means by which they were selected for the study, and any inclusion and exclusion criteria, should be stated. Be explicit about the sampling strategy you adopted, especially if it was other than simple random sampling or a convenience sample. At this stage, restrict yourself to a description of your subjects and how you selected them for the study; what you *did* to them, e.g. in terms of allocation to experimental and control groups, should appear in your description of the research procedure. Incidentally, while the term 'subjects' is wholly appropriate for experimental and most forms of clinical research, when describing survey research you may wish to refer to those whom you studied as 'respondents'.

The next stage is to provide a description of the research design adopted, amplifying on the brief statement already given in the introduction. This gives the reader a good orientation to the overall research strategy you adopted – e.g. a randomized controlled trial, a same-subject longitudinal study, an ethnographic interview study etc. Following this, a detailed, sequential account should be given of the specific steps followed in order to collect the data in the study – as Harris (1986: 38) puts it, this is the part of the methods section 'in which you give a blow-by-blow account of precisely what you said and did to your subjects in the experiment'.

If a standardized, validated instrument was used for data collection – for example the Minnesota Multiphasic Personality Inventory (MMPI) or the Boston Diagnostic Aphasia Examination (BDAE) – it will suffice to give a brief description and refer to a source providing fuller details and specifications. In the case of a piece of hardware, a footnote giving details of the manufacturer is often useful. On the other hand, if an instrument was developed specifically for the present study, you should describe it fully. If a lengthy testing protocol was used, you may prefer to give a brief description in this section and include the full protocol in an appendix. Similarly, it is sometimes helpful to give the full text of a questionnaire in an appendix. On occasions, authors indicate in a footnote that full details of the data collection instrument can be obtained from them on application.

If a pilot study was carried out in order to validate the method of data collection, or to establish a means of calibrating an item of apparatus, this should be described here, together with the results. Lister (1989) recommends that this should be done in the introduction, but as the purpose of a pilot study is to refine data collection procedures, the methods section is its logical home. By the same token, there is no point in holding back the results of the pilot until the results section proper, as they do not form part of the substantive results of the study as a whole. Moreover, this would distort the temporal sequence of the report.

Just as you need to describe the means by which your data were obtained, so you should give an account of how they were analysed, and any statistical procedures employed in the process. This section can conveniently be placed at the end of the methods section, perhaps with its own subheading. Alternatively, it can be located at the beginning of the results section. Opinions differ as to which of these is the optimum location.

Important ethical considerations may attend your choice of research methods (Sim, 1989). You should be prepared to explain and justify how you dealt with these. For example you should give details of the way in which any possible sources of harm to the subjects were monitored, and provide a reasoned justification of any concealment or deception employed. It is particularly important to include details of how informed consent was obtained (Sim, 1986); with some journals, this is a condition of acceptance of a research report. If the approval of a research ethics committee was obtained, this should be stated, but this should be in addition to, not in place of, your own ethical justification of the study.

A difficult question faced when writing the methods section is knowing how much detail you should give. The basic principle is that you should provide sufficient detail for another researcher to replicate your study if he or she chose to. It must be said, however, that this is more easily accomplished in some forms of research than in others. In quantitative research, particularly that employing standardized instrumentation, it may be possible to provide enough detail, in just a few paragraphs, for another worker to repeat your study fairly exactly. In the case of a project involving a long period of participant observation, or a series of lengthy, unstructured interviews, it may not be possible to give all the details that would be required for exact replication. Qualitative research rarely follows rigid, pre-set procedures, but is characterized by more impromptu responses to the immediate demands of the research situation. Often, it is simply impossible to give an exhaustive account of these, and even if such an account were provided, full replication might still not be possible. Another consideration, of course, is the space you have available. As we have already noted, a thesis or dissertation may allow you to describe the research process in minute detail (indeed, your examiners would probably expect this). A journal article, on the other hand, would permit no such luxury. Clearly, all essential facts should be stated, in line with the principle we have already identified, but you should ensure that you do not waste valuable words in a protracted description. O'Connor and Woodford (1978: 22) give the following advice:

> In [the materials and methods] section, change your mental picture of 'the readers' temporarily and regard them as colleagues with research experience similar to your own, so that you do not describe familiar items or procedures in tiresome detail.

Finally, it is worth giving some thought to the order in which you will present information in the methods section. Although we have suggested that you should begin with details of your subjects, you may prefer to follow the advice given by Harris (1986) and start with a description of your research design. Information on your subjects would then follow, prior to a detailed account of your procedure. Rather than follow slavishly any one formula, consider what will be most helpful to the reader. If, for example, the selection of subject was determined by key elements in the research design, it may be appropriate to begin with the latter. On the other hand, if there were no crucial methodological considerations underlying selection, but you wanted to describe your subjects in some detail, you might wish to deal with this at the outset, and then focus the reader's attention fully on the design and procedural issues.

Results

The purpose of this section of a research report is the straightforward reporting of results. As such, it follows the chronological order that we have already observed in the separate sections of the report.

To say that the results are reported is not to say that all the data collected are necessarily presented in their raw form. When dealing with quantitative data, it is in many cases appropriate to reduce them by means of descriptive statistics, and present them in summary form. Do ensure, however, that the summary statistics you choose are suited to your data.

The mean, for example, is an appropriate measure of central tendency for data at the interval or ratio level of measurement, but not usually for ordinal level data (and certainly not for nominal data!). Similarly, standard deviations should be restricted to data that are normally distributed; otherwise a measure of dispersion such as the semi-interquartile range should be employed (consult any comprehensive textbook on statistics for further details; see also chapter 8 for levels of measurement). The right degree of data reduction has to be finely judged:

> A middle course has to be steered between, on the one hand, the presentation of raw and indigestible data which cause reflux rejection and, on the other hand, the temptation to synthesise to such a degree that the original information is lost. (Dudley, 1977: 15)

In addition to summarizing your data by means of descriptive statistics, you will probably need also to analyse them using inferential statistics. In other words, you will wish to indicate whether or not your results are statistically significant (i.e. whether the likelihood of their having come about purely by chance is sufficiently small to be safely ignored). If you haven't already done so at the end of the methods section, this is where you should explain and justify your choice of statistical tests. For a prospective journal article, it is normally not necessary to explain the straightforward aspects of your choice of statistical procedures. However, if you intend to stray from any accepted statistical guidelines (e.g. by applying a parametric test to data which would normally call for a non-parametric test), you should explain why you feel this is permissible. In a thesis or dissertation, however, you may be required to provide a rationale for *all* aspects of your use of inferential statistics.

It is generally considered that statistical significance is the only form of 'significance' with which you should concern yourself in the results section. You should not, as a rule, interpret, discuss or draw any other conclusions from your data at this stage. Rather, you should present your results in an unembellished form, and reserve any commentary for the discussion section, which comes directly after the results section. This is deemed to act as a form of discipline on the researcher, obliging him or her to separate the processes of description and interpretation of the data. By the same token, it allows the reader to evaluate the data prior to reading the researcher's analysis, and thereby reach an independent judgement. It should be said, however, that whereas this is perfectly appropriate for reports adopting a hypothesis-testing approach and dealing primarily with quantitative data, it is not always feasible for other types of research. Imagine, for example, a study into the attitudes and experiences of a group of people with multiple sclerosis in which data were gathered by a series of lengthy, in-depth interviews. There would be no possibility of providing all of the interview transcripts in the report. Necessarily, the extracts presented would be selective, on the basis of the themes they illustrated, the concepts they suggested, and so forth. It would therefore be sensible to discuss these data as they are presented, and thereby convey to the reader the basis on which examples have been selected. To separate presentation from interpretation in a case like this would be bizarre.

Indeed, some writers suggest that a combined results and discussion section is generally to be preferred even when reporting quantitative, experimental research. Sternberg is not convinced by the argument which supports separation of the objective data and the more subjective interpretation, and argues that '[e]ven a slightly skilled writer can interweave data and discussion of the data in a way that makes clear the distinction between the two' (Sternberg, 1988: 55). Whichever approach you favour, you should give due consideration to the specific requirements of individual journals and academic institutions.

A crucial question you must consider is how many results should be presented? Weiss-Lambrou suggests that:

> you must discriminate between those findings which are meaningful, would be of interest and value to the readers, and therefore should be reported and those results which are not relevant, would not be of interest and value to the readers, and consequently, should not be presented. (Weiss-Lambrou, 1989: 42)

This is generally sound advice; there is little point in presenting results which you will not wish subsequently to discuss. It is worth adding, however, that where your research is to appear is an influencing factor here. As you move from a thesis or dissertation, through a report in a scientific journal, to an 'informal' report in a professional magazine, you will need to be increasingly selective in the results that you present.

Finally, in the case of quantitative data, it will readily be apparent that the judicious use of tables and figures will often assist the reader in comprehending your data. See chapter 8 for further details.

Discussion

Kidder and Judd (1986) describe the shape of a research report as resembling an hourglass. In the introduction and literature review, the topic in question is surveyed in fairly broad terms. As you move into the methods and results sections, the focus is necessarily much narrower, as you are concerned only with the specifics of your particular study. The discussion section, however, is where the report begins to broaden again, as you return to more general issues.

The first issue you are likely to want to discuss, however, relates fairly closely to the specific results of your study – was an answer provided to your research question; did your data cause you to retain or reject your hypothesis? Having considered this, you can move on to other, more general aspects of the study:

— possible reasons for any unexpected results;
— the extent to which your findings can be generalized;
— other inferences that can be drawn from the study;
— the way in which your findings fit into the existing knowledge base in this area;
— any shortcomings in the research design or the data collection methods employed;
— the professional relevance of the findings;
— the possibilities for further research in the area which suggest themselves.

Clearly, many of the questions you will be addressing will have been touched upon in the introduction, and there will be close links between the two sections. In particular, you will need to return to some of the key sources discussed in the review of the literature. However, whereas previously you had considered the work of others in terms of planning your own study and establishing your research question, you will now be discussing these sources in the light of your own newly-acquired findings.

When discussing the inferences to be drawn from your results, your primary focus should be on those inferences that relate specifically to your research question or hypothesis and are directly supported by the data. However, this is not to say that you cannot also discuss inferences that are only *suggested* by your findings, or which relate to other research questions which, with hindsight, your data might have answered better. The important thing is to make it absolutely clear that you are engaging in post hoc speculation, and that you are not making claims fully supported by the findings obtained.

The rôle of the discussion section, then, may be summed up as providing an answer to the question 'what does it all show?'

Conclusion

The conclusion is usually a very brief part of the research paper, which serves principally to round off your discussion (indeed, in some instances it may not be a section in its own right; its function may be fulfilled by the final paragraph or two in the discussion section). Here, you should highlight the principal findings of your study and the most noteworthy conclusions to be drawn from them. In other words, think about the main points that you wish the reader to come away with after having read your report, and outline these clearly and concisely. Resist the temptation to provide a summary of the whole report – that is merely to duplicate the function of the abstract.

The conclusion is followed by the acknowledgements (if any) and the list of references. Those whom you should acknowledge include friends or colleagues who gave advice on the study (but did not participate in it directly), staff who provided apparatus or other material help, and individuals or institutions who afforded facilities or financial support. Weiss-Lambrou (1989) suggests that it is not necessary to acknowledge those, such as secretaries, whose normal duties required them to be involved in your study. O'Connor and Woodford (1978: 25) recommend that you ensure 'that all those you thank agree to having their help recognized and that they approve the form in which you acknowledge it'. The principal reason for seeking approval from those whom you intend to name is that their inclusion in the acknowledgements may be perceived as an endorsement of the contents of the paper.

The listing of references was considered in chapter 6.

Stylistic and grammatical considerations

A question which can cause some concern is which tense to use when writing a research report. Table 7.1 gives some guidelines, based on the recommendations of Day (1989) and Lister (1989). The alternation of tense between your own work and that of other workers whom you cite may strike you as rather odd. However, Day (1989) explains the underlying reasons convincingly. Once published, others' work has been accepted by their professional peers (through the process of peer review referred to earlier), and it passes into the knowledge base. This is acknowledged by stating their findings and conclusions in the present tense (what they actually *did* to gain these results stays in the past tense, of course). However, your own findings are, at the time of writing the report, yet to be so accepted, and you recognize this fact by using the past tense; i.e. you're saying 'this is what happened (in this particular case)', not 'this is what happens (as a general rule or tendency)'.

The following quotation illustrates the use of the active voice (where a verb describes someone or something *acting*) and the passive voice (where it describes someone or something *being acted upon*):

Next, we asked [active voice] each subject to breathe in deeply before exhaling as hard and fast as possible. At the beginning

Table 7.1 *Use of tense in different sections of the research report*

Section	Tense required	Example
Introduction	Present	'Occupational stress *is* an under-researched topic in speech and language therapy.'
Literature Review	Past for the work of others; present for their results	'Klein and Denby (1989) *studied* stress levels among mid-career therapists, and *showed* that stress *varies* with clinical specialty and *is* related to length of experience.'
Method	Past	'We *administered* two follow-up questionnaires at intervals of eight weeks.'
Results	Past	'Therapists working with severely dysphasic patients *displayed* a distinct pattern of stressors.'
Discussion	Past for your work; present for the work of others or your own previously published work	'We found that most respondents *relied* on peer support to deal with potentially stressful situations. This is in agreement with the study by James et al. (1987), whose results suggest that therapists *adopt* this strategy in preference to more formal mechanisms.'
		'In an earlier study (Dale et al., 1987) we found that these therapists *display* a distinct pattern of stressors.'

of this forced expiration, the switch on the spirometer was activated [passive voice].

Despite a traditional preference for the passive voice in scientific writing, there is a considerable body of opinion nowadays maintaining that the active voice is clearer and more direct, and therefore to be preferred (Kidder and Judd, 1986; Lister, 1989; Day, 1989). It is certainly more concise than the passive voice, and equates more closely with spoken English. However, as the passage above illustrates, the two can be effectively used together.

Closely linked to this issue is the use of the first person, as opposed to the third person. On those occasions when the active voice was used, traditional scientific English mandated the third person: 'The researchers ensured that subjects were adequately briefed as to the range of responses required.' However, it is now often acceptable to use the first person: 'We ensured that subjects . . .' In fact, there are occasions when the first person is distinctly preferable. If, for example, you are giving an account of a piece of qualitative research in which your rôle as a researcher has theoretical or methodological implications for the study, referring to yourself in the third person can be inappropriate, as the following example suggests:

> As the interviews progressed, the researcher found that her own emotional responses were increasingly hard to ignore. The social situation of the respondents frequently elicited feelings of pity and anger in the interviewer. The researcher was thus placed in an uncomfortable dilemma.

However, as we have repeatedly indicated, you will generally have to conform to the stylistic requirements of the publication for which you are writing, or the institution to which you are presenting your work. Note, however, that in research reports it is very unusual to address the reader in the second person (e.g. 'you will see from the results in Table 5 . . .').

In many forms of written English, it is considered good style to make use of synonyms, so as to avoid overusing a particular word. In scientific writing, however, this should be done with caution, so as not to introduce ambiguity. If, in an account of a study into occupational stress, you refer initially to 'stressors', and then later talk about 'sources of stress' or 'stressful stimuli', you may give the reader the impression that you intend these items to refer to different factors or phenomena. It may be felt, for example, that 'sources of stress' are meant to refer to situational or environmental factors, whereas 'stressful stimuli' are interactive factors. Similarly, if you use a thesaurus, do so judiciously, with due regard to subtle differences of meaning between apparent synonyms.

If you are submitting a paper to an American publication, you should ensure that you adopt appropriate terminology (e.g. 'physical therapy' rather than 'physiotherapy', 'chronic obstructive pulmonary disease (COPD)' rather than 'chronic obstructive airways disease (COAD)') and spelling ('center' rather than 'centre', 'behavioral' rather than 'behavioural'). An American dictionary, such as that compiled by Ehrlich et al. (1980), should be consulted in cases of uncertainty.

Finally, a word or two about jargon. Given that your research is likely to be conducted within a closely focused topic, you will probably be drawn into an area of specialized vocabulary which may be quite specific to that topic. How should you handle this specialist terminology? On the one hand, you might feel that it would assist your prospective readers if you were to translate some of these technical terms into those which are more current in professional parlance. In the process, however, you are at risk of losing some of the specificity of meaning of the original term, and you may make it difficult for readers to relate your study to other work which may have retained the specialist vocabulary. On the other hand, if you retain all the specialist terms, this may make your report off-putting and laborious to read. This is where it is important to consider your intended readership. The degree of familiarity of your readers with the technical vocabulary will differ, depending on whether you are publishing in a professional journal aimed at generalists within a given profession, one devoted to specialists, or one whose readership is multidisciplinary, such as *Clinical Rehabilitation* or the *Journal of Allied Health*. Whatever approach you adopt in relation to this question, our earlier advice to provide explicit working definitions of key terms still applies.

Conclusion

Like all pieces of writing, a scientific paper requires careful planning and attention to detail, and it is particularly important to consider the accepted conventions that govern the structure and composition of such papers. However, you should not follow these too slavishly; if there are good reasons for departing from the traditional format you should not hesitate to do so. Above all, you should think of what the reader, unfamiliar with your research, needs to know about it, and construct your report accordingly.

Chapter

8

The Use of Graphics

This chapter will consider the ways in which written text, especially that concerned with imparting quantitative data, can be enhanced and augmented by the graphic presentation of information. General guidelines will be given as to the principles underlying successful graphics, and the strengths and weaknesses of various graphic forms will be addressed.

Enhancing written text with visual aids

The cliché that 'one picture is worth a thousand words' has an element of truth in it; there are a number of ways in which the written word can be assisted by visual aids. These include such things as tables, graphs, photographs, line drawings and flow diagrams. Although there are many forms of graphics, in publishing vocabulary they can be divided into two: *tables* fall into a category of their own, while all the remainder constitute what are known as *figures*. In this chapter, however, we will not deal with these media under these two headings; it is perhaps more helpful to consider first those means of visually representing quantitative information, and then those to do with more pictorial forms of information. Before moving onto specific issues, however, it is important to consider some of the general principles underlying the use of graphics.

Broadly speaking, visual aids serve to enrich two aspects of your writing: its appearance and its intelligibility. The relative importance of these two factors will depend on the writing medium in question. To consider the matter of appearance first, there is no doubt that pages of text unrelieved by any form of illustrative matter can be forbidding, or at best unwelcoming, for the reader, especially if there is little use of headings to break the flow of text. If you are writing for a newspaper, or a professional magazine such as *Therapy Weekly*, the judicious use of illustrations – even if only a photograph of the author! – can serve to attract the reader's attention. This may be particularly important in the case of a multidisciplinary readership, where it is often necessary to stimulate readers to look at material in fields other than their own. In such a medium, visual aids are not necessarily indispensable to the content of the article concerned. In a piece concerned with patterns of referral to speech and language therapy, a photograph of a therapist and a patient at work may not convey any information over and above that contained in the text; its function is to enhance the impact of the message contained in the text and make it more pleasing to the eye.

On the other hand, if you consider a paper in a professional journal, a piece of research written up in a thesis or dissertation, or an undergraduate coursework assignment, the rôle of non-textual material is different. Although graphs, tables and illustrations will often do much to assist the appearance of the text, they are never there for just that reason. They will each have a distinct rôle to play in terms of the content of the paper, and the author's meaning is not just enhanced by such visual aids, it largely depends upon them. In other words, we are more concerned here with the notion of intelligibility, whereas in less academic media the question of appearance is more at stake.

Clearly, various textual and non-textual forms each have their own advantages and disadvantages. These are concisely summed up as follows:

> A text can explain, interpret, and evaluate; a table can provide exact comparisons and supporting evidence; and a chart can demonstrate, communicate at a glance with force, conviction, and appeal, and possibly disclose relationships that might otherwise pass unnoticed. (Schmid and Schmid, 1979: 7)

We will return to some more specific considerations connected with the use of graphics after looking at some of the forms they can take.

Displaying quantitative information

Before we can proceed to look at specific means of displaying quantitative information, it is vital to understand the forms in which it can be expressed, as these often have a direct bearing on the sort of visual display that should be chosen. The most important subdivision of quantitative information is expressed in terms of 'levels of measurement', of which there are four.

Measurement at the *nominal* level is the most basic, and simply consists in assigning cases to different categories according to type; there is no difference in degree or magnitude. Place of birth, occupation, sex, hair colour, marital status and political affiliation are all examples of nominal measurements. A nominal scale consisting of two categories (e.g. sex) is known as a dichotomous scale.

Data on an *ordinal* scale go one stage further than those measured at the nominal level. Not only are cases assigned to various categories, but these categories can be placed in some sort of hierarchy according to degree or magnitude. Examples of such ranked categories would include social class, responses on a Likert scale (e.g. strongly agree, agree, no opinion, disagree, strongly disagree), and professional grade as a therapist (e.g. junior, senior II, senior I etc.). You will notice that, although we know that one category is either higher or lower than another, we do not know precisely by how much. We cannot say whether, for example, the difference on a Likert scale between 'strongly agree' and 'agree' is the same as, greater than, or less than the difference between 'no opinion' and 'disagree'.

Measurement at the *interval* level makes up this deficiency in an ordinal scale. Here, we know not only that the points on a scale are in an order of degree or magnitude, but also that they are equally far apart. That is, 'numerically equal distances on interval scales represent equal distances in the property being measured' (Kerlinger 1973: 437). Thus, on an IQ scale, we know that the difference between somebody with an IQ of 140 and somebody with one of 150 is the same as the difference between somebody with an IQ of 120 and somebody with one of 130.

A *ratio* scale has the same properties as an interval scale, except that whereas an interval scale has an arbitrary zero point, a ratio scale has an absolute, or 'true', zero point. On a ratio scale, such as weight or height, zero does in fact mean no weight or no height. However, in the case of IQ, which is on an interval scale, an IQ of 0 does not represent a total absence of intelligence. To clarify this distinction further, compare the Celsius (interval) and Kelvin (ratio) scales of temperature. The freezing point of water, which is 0 degrees Celsius, is arbitrary, as there is still molecular movement and thus some degree of heat. In contrast, 0 degrees Kelvin is absolute zero, which is a true zero as it represents total absence of heat. Table 8.1 summarizes the properties of different levels of measurement, and illustrates the fact that one level of measurement can always be reduced to a lower level, but that certain information is lost in the process.

Finally, a word or two needs to be said about the distinction between discrete and continuous data. With *discrete* data, it is either not possible to interpose categories between those given, or else such interpolation cannot be performed precisely or meaningfully. The number of children in a family is therefore on a discrete scale; there are no possibilities between, say, one child and two. Alternatively, take a five point ordinal pain scale, where 5 represents excruciating pain, 4 severe pain, 3 moderate pain and so forth. While there

Table 8.1 *Descriptive properties of different levels of measurement*

Level	Category	Rank	Equal interval	True zero
Nominal	√			
Ordinal	√	√		
Interval	√	√	√	
Ratio	√	√	√	√

obviously are possible intensities of pain between any two adjacent points on this scale, it is not possible to interpolate them; rather, another scale with more scale points would be required. In the case of *continuous* data, however, it is possible to interpolate points between those actually represented on the scale – age, height and weight are examples. Babbie (1989: 373) expresses the difference well when he remarks that a continous variable 'increases steadily in tiny fractions instead of jumping from category to category as does a discrete variable.'

The relevance of the various levels of measurement and the distinction between discrete and continuous data will become clearer when considering specific methods of displaying quantitative data.

Pie charts

The pie chart, a variant of which was first developed by Florence Nightingale (Reid and Boore, 1987), is illustrated in Figure 8.1.

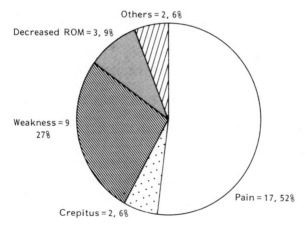

Figure 8.1 *Pie chart representing the frequency of shoulder problems among full-time participants in sport, based on a sample of 33 participants. From: Lo Y.P.C., Hsu Y.C.S., Chan K.M. (1990) Epidemiology of shoulder impingement in upper arm sports events.* British Journal of Sports Medicine *24, 173–177, reproduced with permission of the publisher.*

This is a visual aid which you might wish to use for data on a nominal scale. Specifically, it illustrates the percentages of a set of data which fall into various categories – each percentage point is represented by 3.6 degrees of the circle. As demonstrated in Figure 8.1, the numerical data on which the percentages are based can (and usually should) be given in addition to the percentage values, but not instead of them. To improve the clarity of the pie chart, each segment can be shaded or hatched in a different manner; this also allows the segments to be identified by means of a key, rather than being labelled directly, which can clutter the chart. The success of a pie chart to some extent depends upon the number and size of the segments. As Cormack (1984: 50) indicates:

> If many items are included, for example in excess of ten, the large number of relatively small parts will be difficult to distinguish from each other. Similarly, as parts become smaller and represent tiny percentages, 1% for example, it becomes very difficult to indicate to the reader what such parts represent.

Conversely, there is little point in using a pie chart for less than three segments, as no greater clarity is likely to be obtained than by simply stating the percentage in question.

Two or more pie charts can be used together, to convey information about two or more sets of data. In this case, the charts can be presented in proportionate sizes, so that if one data set is twice as large as another, its pie chart can be correspondingly larger. Leach (1988) is critical of pie charts, however, as he claims that people find it hard to judge area accurately. It is certainly fair to say that 'three-dimensional' pie charts, which require judgements not just of area but of volume as well, should be avoided, despite their visual appeal and the ease with which computer software can produce them.

Because the segments making up the chart have no particular order to them, a pie chart is less suitable for ordinal data. However, it is often sensible to arrange segments in order of size. A pie chart is generally read from the 'twelve o'clock position', and segments can be displayed in ascending or descending order of size from this point (note that Figure 8.1 does not adopt this strategy).

Bar charts

These can be used for nominal data, but are especially suitable for ordinal data, in that it is easy to display categories in rank order. The bars are generally arranged vertically – i.e. on the horizontal axis (sometimes referred to as the abscissa, or x axis). On occasions the bars may be horizontally disposed – i.e. on the vertical axis (sometimes known as the ordinate, or y axis) as in Figure 8.2. Some sources, such as Schmid and Schmid (1979), refer to the former as column charts, and reserve the term bar chart for the latter. Note that the bars in Figure 8.2 are not contiguous; this is to represent the fact that nominal or ordinal data are discrete, not continuous.

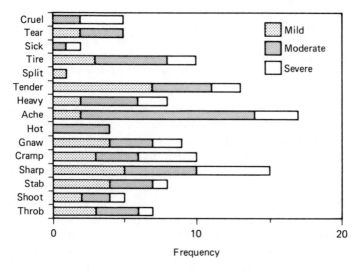

Figure 8.2 *Descriptions of pain by 23 subjects with painful knee disorders. The divided bars indicate the intensity of the pain described. Note that subjects frequently gave more than one description of their pain, and therefore the total frequency count is greater than 23. Figure by courtesy of Jackie Waterfield.*

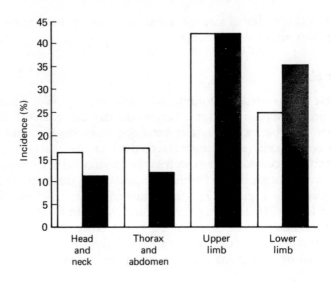

Figure 8.3   *Anatomical location of injury to motor cyclists: comparison of the incidence on the race track to that on the public road. Shaded bars = public road, unshaded bars = race track. From: Chapman M.A.S., Oni J. (1991) Motor racing accidents at Brands Hatch, 1988/9.* British Journal of Sports Medicine *25, 121–123. Reproduced with permission of the publisher.*

In the example shown in Figure 8.3, the bars arranged on the horizontal axis represent the various categories, while the scale on the vertical axis shows the frequency (i.e. the number of cases in each category). Although the frequency scale is usually given in absolute numbers, it is perfectly permissible to present it as a percentage scale (as it is in Figure 8.3).

When frequencies are displayed against the vertical axis, the scale should start at zero and should be uninterrupted. In this case, the reader is usually asked to make comparative judgements (i.e. assess relative frequencies), and to use a truncated or interrupted scale would distort such judgements. For example a bar which is twice the height of another would represent a frequency which is less than twice as great. However, when displaying variate information (i.e. specific values of a variable rather than the number of cases which lie at such values), this rule can sometimes be bent. For example you may wish to display values which lie between 120 and 135; this would tend to require very tall bars. A way round this is either to begin the scale at, say, 100, or to use a scale break (i.e. the scale begins at zero, but a portion of it is removed and the remainder of the scale is closed up; the excised portion is represented by two parallel lines drawn through the scale). This produces a chart of a more manageable size, though the relative heights of the bars may still be misleading to the inattentive reader, and this strategy should therefore be used cautiously. When a scale break is used, it should be shown on both the scale and the bars (Schmid and Schmid, 1979).

On occasions, the height of the bars may represent not a specific value, but the mean of a group of values (note that this is strictly speaking a misuse of bar charts, but it is nonetheless fairly common practice). For example each bar might represent a different infectious disease, and its height might indicate the mean duration of the incubation period in days. In such a case, it is often useful to indicate the dispersion of the figures from which the mean was calculated. Usually, this is done by indicating one standard deviation either side of the mean, and this can be accomplished by thin vertical lines above and below the bars.

Grouped bar charts can also be used. Here, each category can be subdivided into two or more sub-categories. For example if the categories represented age bands, each of these age bands could contain two bars, to represent males and females. In this case the bars within each category would be differently shaded or hatched, so as to distinguish them clearly from one another, and would be contiguous (though they would be separated from neighbouring pairs of grouped bars in categories on each side). An example of a grouped bar chart can be seen in Figure 8.3. To save space, the bars within each category can be made to overlap partially; this is known as a stacked bar chart. An alternative strategy is to subdivide individual bars; this is adopted in Figure 8.2.

The comments made earlier as to the number of segments in a pie chart are applicable to bar charts; as a general rule, a chart which contains less than three bars is unlikely to have much greater impact than the corresponding absolute figures.

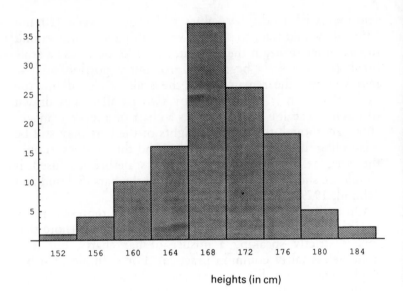

Figure 8.4   *Histogram showing the distribution of heights of a random sample of individuals (hypothetical data). The figures on the horizontal axis represent the midpoints of the class intervals (e.g. 160 = 158.5 – 162.5). Figure courtesy of Dr Mark Muldoon.*

Histograms

A histogram (Figure 8.4) is like a bar chart in appearance, but has a number of important differences. The principal of these is that the rectangles in a histogram are contiguous; this is to reflect the fact that a histogram is used for continuous data, while, as we noted, a bar chart is used for discrete data.

Note that some scales, such as age bands, are strictly speaking discrete, but have an underlying continuity; a histogram is appropriate here. Social class, however, is an ordinal scale which is wholly discrete, and a histogram would be unsuitable in this case.

Another difference between the two forms of chart is that in a histogram the order of the rectangles is fixed by the continuous data being presented; in a bar chart displaying nominal categories the order in which the bars appear is largely immaterial. Finally, while a bar chart can be displayed either vertically or horizontally, the rectangles in a histogram should nearly always be vertical.

Frequency polygons

A frequency polygon (Figure 8.5) is a form of line chart. A line chart (often referred to simply as a 'graph') is exactly what its name would suggest – a two-dimensional chart on which a series of points are connected by a line. Like a histogram, a frequency polygon plots a continuous variable on the horizontal axis against frequency on the vertical axis.

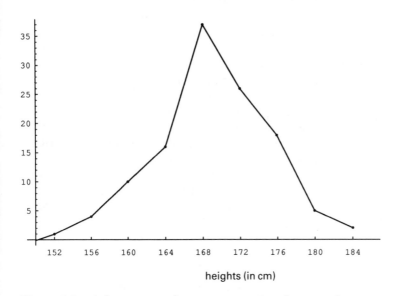

heights (in cm)

Figure 8.5 *A frequency polygon, representing the same data as the histogram in Figure 8.4. Figure courtesy of Dr Mark Muldoon.*

Indeed, frequency polygons and histograms are interconvertible, such that data which can be displayed as one can also be displayed as the other. The difference is that whereas a histogram plots a frequency distribution by a series of bars, a polygon does so by means of a continuous line. Such a line makes it easier to interpolate between data points, and to this extent a polygon is to be preferred to a histogram. However, it is sometimes valuable to group individual data points into class intervals, such as age bands. In this case, the bars in a histogram represent these intervals much more clearly than a polygon. A frequency polygon can always be superimposed on a histogram by joining the midpoints of the top of each rectangle with a line. Moreover, a number of different frequency polygons can readily be superimposed on one another (though this is much more difficult with histograms).

Stem-and-leaf plots

The stem-and leaf plot is an extremely useful, but rather neglected, means of presenting interval or ratio data. It has the particular merit of providing a pictorial image of a data set without significant loss of information. It is worth explaining this in some detail. Suppose, for example, you wanted to display the marks obtained by a group of 60 students on an examination, and that the range of marks was from 32 to 81. On a bar chart, your vertical axis would be the number of students (frequency), and the bars on the horizontal axis would represent a discrete scale corresponding to the possible scores (from 1 to 100, assuming the examination carried a maximum possible mark of 100). It should be clear that to allocate a bar to each possible score would produce a very wide chart that would be very hard to interpret. In order to gain a more meaningful picture of the data, the scores could be compacted by placing them into equal bands, or class intervals (e.g. 0 – 4, 5–9, 10–14, 15–19, 20–24 etc.). Thus, the original scale could be grouped into categories which would highlight the key features of the distribution of the data, yet produce a more economical figure. However, in the process the individual data points would be lost; you would know that there were, let us say, six students with scores between 41 and 45, but you would not be able to tell how many students, if any, obtained a score of, for example, 43. In a stem-and-leaf plot, such as that shown in Figure 8.6, a higher level of information is preserved; the shape of the distribution is presented in a similar way to a histogram, but the specific data points are not lost in the process.

```
0*  |
0.  |
1*  |
1.  |
2*  |
2.  |
3*  |  23
3.  |  577
4*  |  2334
4.  |  59
5*  |  0112333
5.  |  56677788899
6*  |  001233344
6.  |  556666788
7*  |  1112234
7.  |  5688
8*  |  11
8.  |
9*  |
9.  |
```

Figure 8.6 *Stem-and-leaf plot of the marks of 60 students in an examination marked out of 100. Stem unit = 10.*

Those figures to the left of the vertical line represent the 'stem', and they are the class intervals. In this case, we have class intervals of five, and these are presented according to the following convention:

2* = 20–24
2. = 25–29

3* = 30–34
3. = 35–39 etc.

The figures to the right of the vertical line are the 'leaves', and these units are one tenth the value of the stem units. The leaves represent the specific data points. Accordingly, the leaves corresponding to the stems marked '7*' and '7.' can be expressed in terms of the original raw scores: 71, 71, 71, 72, 72, 73, 74, 75, 76, 78, 78. Note that a declaration must be made of the stem units, to make it clear that one stem unit is 10, rather than, for example, 1000, 100 or 0.1.

There are a number of variations that can be performed on the basic stem-and-leaf plot. The scale of the stem can be either compressed or expanded. In the latter case, each stem can be made to represent two units rather than five, thus:

2* = 20–21
2t = 22–23
2f = 24–25
2s = 26–27
2. = 28–29

(the 't' stands for 'twos and threes', the 'f' for 'fours and fives', and the 's' for 'sixes and sevens'). In addition, two frequency distributions can be plotted on the same stem, one on either side (the examination scores could be plotted with males students to the right of the stem, and female students to the left, for example).

In both histograms and stem-and-leaf plots, care must be taken in choosing the most appropriate number of class intervals 'as too many will reduce the number of values in each one, emphasizing minor fluctuations, and too few will obscure the true variability of the data' (Brown and Beck, 1990: 12).

A more detailed discussion of stem-and-leaf plots can be found in Marsh (1988).

Scattergrams

A scattergram (or scatterplot) is a means of displaying the relationship between two continuous variables, where a value on both variables can be assigned to each case in a set of data. Figure 8.7 shows the relationship between total white blood cell (WBC) count and total granulocyte count in 55 patients (cases). Each case is plotted at the point at which its WBC count intersects its granulocyte count. In this way, a visual impression of the degree of association between the two variables can be obtained, and a regression line (the dotted line in Figure 8.7) can be drawn to show the linear relationship. Because variate information is concerned here, rather than frequencies, it is permissible not to start the axes at zero in order to produce a more compact figure.

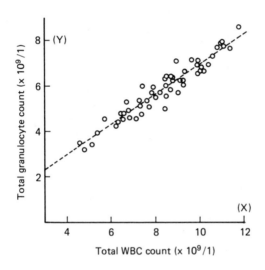

Figure 8.7   *Scattergram representing the relationship between total white blood cell count and total granulocyte count in 55 patients with malignant bronchial lesions. The broken line indicates the regression line. From: Strike P.W. (1991)* Statistical Methods in Laboratory Medicine. *Oxford: Butterworth-Heinemann, p 242, reproduced with permission of the publisher.*

If the two variables represent an independent (predictor) and a dependent (outcome) variable, the former is conventionally plotted on the horizontal axis and the latter on the vertical axis.

Time-series charts

Another variety of line chart or graph is the time-series chart – sometimes referred to as a 'fever chart', after its familiar use in recording changes in body temperature (Holmes, 1984). Here, an interval or ratio variable (e.g. expenditure on splinting materials, number of outpatient referrals) is plotted on the vertical axis, and the horizontal axis represents time in appropriate intervals. This allows the examination of trends over time. More than one line can be plotted on the same chart, as illustrated in Figure 8.8.

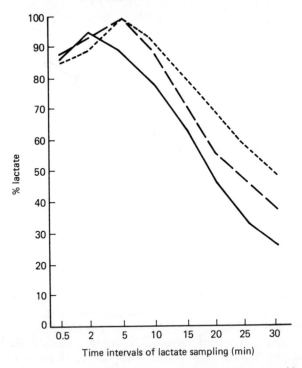

Figure 8.8 *A time-series chart showing blood lactate profiles in various recovery regimes, following exhaustive arm exercise. Results are expressed as a percentage of mean maximum lactate values. The different lines represent the three different recovery regimens. From: Baker S.J., King N. (1991) Lactic acid recovery profiles following exhaustive arm exercise on a canoeing ergometer.* British Journal of Sports Medicine 25, 165–167, *reproduced with permission of the publisher.*

Tables

A table is simply a means of presenting data by categorizing two or more variables against each other in rows and columns. Each point of intersection of a row and a column creates a 'cell' into which data can be entered. A simple table is shown in Table 8.2. The cells in this table contain quantitative data, but a table can also include symbols (e.g. the ticks in Table 8.1 earlier in this chapter) or words (as in Table 7.1 in the previous chapter).

Table 8.2   *Attitudes of occupational therapists of different grades to a restructuring of therapy services within a district health authority (hypothetical data). Figures shown in parentheses are percentages.*

| | Occupational therapy staff | | | | |
	Junior	*Senior II*	*Senior I*	*Head III & above*	*TOTAL*
In favour	56 (75)	24 (66)	14 (67)	5 (50)	99 (70)
Against	14 (19)	10 (28)	7 (33)	4 (40)	35 (25)
Don't know	4 (6)	2 (6)	0 (0)	1 (10)	7 (5)
TOTAL	74	36	21	10	141

The construction and use of figures and tables

There are a number of general principles which govern the way in which figures and tables are constructed and utilized.

It is generally accepted that data given in the text of a report should not be repeated in a table, and vice versa (Currier, 1975; Leach, 1988). Rather, a choice should be made as to which is the most effective means of presentation. However, some authorities maintain that a chart or graph can legitimately contain information that has also been given in textual or tabular form. The rationale for this is as follows:

> Graphs should always be regarded as subsidiary aids to the intelligence and not as the *evidence* of associations or trends. That evidence must be largely drawn from the statistical tables themselves. It follows that graphs are an unsatisfactory *substitute* for statistical tables. (Hill and Hill, 1991: 53, original emphasis)

Day, on the other hand, generally recommends choosing between graphs and tables, and suggests that 'your choice might relate to whether you want to impart to readers exact numerical values or simply a picture of the trend or shape of the data' (Day, 1989: 65). Similarly, Chapman and Mahon (1986) point out that charts are generally to be preferred to tables when you wish to emphasize comparisons; the underlying principle, they suggest, is that charts should be used to display data for demonstration purposes, but not for reference purposes.

Whether a table or a figure is being used, it should fulfil a goal that text alone cannot attain. The information to be conveyed to the reader in graphic form must gain in clarity or meaningfulness as compared with textual exposition; if it does not, the visual aid becomes a distraction rather than an aid to comprehension. In particular, do not feel that all quantitative data in a report or other piece of work need be given in the same form; depending on the nature of the various sets of data, tubular presentation may be appropriate on some occasions, bar charts or histograms at other times, and verbal description in yet other instances.

Tables and figures should be intelligible independently of the text. Readers may have to resort to the text to appreciate the *significance* of the table or figure, but they should be able to interpret its *meaning* as it stands. For this reason, a sufficiently informative legend should be supplied. Similarly, you should ensure that all units are given and all scales fully labelled. A common error in respect of this is to state a rate without specifying the base on which it is measured, e.g. whether the incidence of a particular condition is per cent, per thousand or per million (Hill and Hill, 1991).

Observe two cardinal principles when constructing graphics – clarity and economy. Try to ensure that the medium does not distort or obstruct the message. Tufte suggests that one of the principles of what he calls 'graphical excellence' is that of giving 'the viewer the greatest number of ideas in the shortest time with the least ink in the smallest space' (Tufte, 1983: 51).

In addition to the above general principles, there are a few other specific points which should be made in relation to tables and figures:

(1) If possible, try to construct tables with horizontal lines only, as this is insisted on by some publishers.

(2) Use abbreviations with care and due regard to your target publication. Will your intended readership realize that 'SEM' stands for 'standard error of the mean'? It is good practice to explain such abbreviations in the legend or in a key, even if you have already done so in the text.

(3) When selecting the size of lettering in figures, bear in mind the eventual size of the figure after possible reduction.

(4) Consider also the dimensions of the figure as a whole. In particular, bear in mind that a published figure will usually have to occupy the width of either one or two columns of text. Tall, thin figures are especially difficult to accommodate in this respect.

(5) Consider the use of different type faces in tables. Hill and Hill (1991) suggest that absolute numbers and percentages can usefully be distinguished in this way, e.g. by presenting the latter in italics. Similarly, figures that are statistically significant can be given in bold type. Make sure, of course, that you explain the meaning of such refinements!

(6) In tables, do not align numerals at the left; rather, align decimal points. Hence, this is correct:

$$12.01$$
$$102.67$$
$$7.60$$

whereas this is not:

$$12.01$$
$$102.67$$
$$7.60$$

(7) Always display decimals to the same number of places. It would be incorrect, in the example above, to give the last value simply as 7.6; the reason for this is that it tells the reader that the second decimal place has not been rounded up or down. Incidentally, rounding can be an effective means of conveying the amount of measurement error you feel may be present; if you suspect there is approximately a 10 per cent measurement error, you may wish to reflect this by eliminating the last decimal place in your actual measurements.

(8) If you have a long column of figures in a table, it will be easier to read if the figures are grouped into blocks of five.

(9) When constructing graphs, remember that the angle of the graph line is determined by the relationship of the scale on the vertical axis to that on the horizontal axis; if one of these is unduly compressed or expanded relative to the other, this can have the effect of artificially flattening or accentuating the slope of the graph line.

(10) Be wary of making use of potentially gimmicky features such as three-dimensional bar charts or pie charts. Although these can be visually impressive, they rarely enhance, but frequently undermine, the intelligibility of a figure. In this connection, note Tufte's remarks: 'Graphical displays should . . . induce the viewer to think about the substance rather than about methodology, graphic design, the technology of graphic production, or something else' (Tufte, 1983: 13).

(11) When submitting figures for publication, ensure that the legends are on a separate sheet, and not on the figures themselves; this is because the legends will be typeset, whereas the figures will be photographically reproduced. Also, ensure that there is a textual reference to each figure, as it may not be possible to place the figure in immediate juxtaposition to the piece of text to which it relates.

(12) If you have more than one line on a single graph, distinguish these clearly (for example, by making one a continuous line, another a broken line, and another a dotted line, as in Figure 8.8).

(13) If you want readers to compare two or more tables or figures, try to construct them to a standard format; in particular, ensure that axes are not arbitrarily transposed between charts showing similar information, and retain the order of listing in tables unless there are good reasons for doing otherwise. Be consistent in your use of capitals and lower-case in labelling – in relation to this, O'Connor and Woodford (1978) recommend lower-case for whole words.

(14) Above all, observe what Tufte (1983) calls 'graphical integrity'. Ensure that you do not give a false or misleading impression of your data by the use of techniques which distort their true value. Some of the features already noted – such as scale breaks on frequency scales, unduly compressed or expanded axes, and the use of

three-dimensional techniques – can easily have this effect. Huff (1973) and Tufte (1983) provide illuminating examples of misleading graphics.

Displaying pictorial and similar information

Not all the information that can be conveyed in graphic form is quantitative. Figures can be used to convey pictorial images, or to portray processes or conceptual relationships in diagrammatic form.

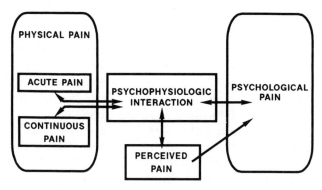

Figure 8.9 *A flow chart diagram illustrating interaction between physiological and psychological elements in the perception of pain. From: Königová R. (1992) The psychological problems of burned patients. The Rudy Hermans Lecture 1991. Burns 18, 189–199, reproduced with permission of the publisher.*

Flow charts

Various sorts of processes or interactions can be illustrated by means of a flow chart or variant thereof, as in Figure 8.9. Similar diagrams, known as decision-structure tables (Enrick, 1972), can be valuable in portraying diagnostic algorithms or explaining clinical management decisions.

Line drawings and photographs

The use of these media is largely self-explanatory, but a few remarks as to their relative pros and cons are perhaps in order.

The chief advantage of a photograph is, of course, that it has greater verisimilitude than a line drawing. For example if you wished to illustrate some aspect of therapist–patient communication, a photograph would probably convey a more convincing image (provided it wasn't too 'posed') than a line drawing; the latter might have a rather artificial or idealized air about it. On the other hand, a line drawing may do a better job of illustrating a therapeutic technique, as certain details can be emphasized, and others de-emphasized, in order to clarify the essential points of the manoeuvre (e.g. Figure 8.10). Additionally, it is easier to add explanatory symbols and devices, such as arrows or dotted lines, to line drawings than to photographs. If you are a competent artist, you can generate line drawings at minimal cost, whereas some expense is always incurred in producing photographic illustrations. Moreover, inexpert line drawings (known as 'roughs') can be refashioned by a professional artist, whereas it is not always possible to retake photographs, not least because the 'live' subject matter may no longer be available.

If you decide to use photographs, it is advisable to employ the services of a professional photographer, who will be able to advise on the appropriate type, format and speed of film, and will arrange suitable lighting conditions. Most publishers prefer black-and-white glossy prints, large enough to permit reduction to about half their size during photographic reproduction. If you decide to do your own photography, Wells (1983) and Hines (1987) offer some useful advice.

Some publishers will reproduce colour photographs, but the author may have to bear the cost of this. Make sure to check whether the publisher prefers prints or transparencies. Although colour can always be reproduced as black and white – and may therefore seem to be a way of keeping your options open – this is a misguided strategy, as the results are always inferior to original black-and-white photographs. You should, in any case, give careful thought to the use of colour in any form of illustration, especially in academic or scientific writing. Although colour can be eye-catching, you should ask if it is serving a purpose of which black and white is not capable. If not, it may hinder, rather than facilitate, the message you are trying to put across. There is no merit in

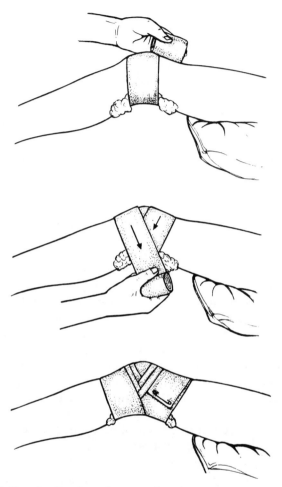

Figure 8.10 *Application of a crêpe bandage to the knee. From: Thomson A., Skinner A., Piercy J. (1991)* Tidy's Physiotherapy *12th edn. Oxford: Butterworth-Heinemann, p 47, reproduced with permission of the publisher.*

making a figure more aesthetically pleasing if in the process its substance is undermined. Bear in mind also, from a practical point of view, that you may be required to submit several copies of a piece of work to a journal or an educational institution; photocopies of coloured originals are very expensive. The various uses of colour in charts and diagrams are illustrated in Holmes (1984).

When producing line drawings, it is important to acquire drawing pens of professional quality, rather than everyday felt tip pens and the like. Equal care should go into the choice of paper; you should opt for fine grain paper or card, again of professional quality (a supplier of artists' materials will give appropriate advice). Shading and hatching can present particular problems. Large areas of shading are likely to appear uneven if done in ink and by hand; this can be overcome by cutting special film (e.g. Rubylith) to shape and attaching it over the area to be shaded. Hatching lines should not be too faint, or they will not show up if they have to be reduced. Similarly, if lines are too close together, they tend to fill in when reproduced, and resemble shading.

Line drawings and, particularly, photographs need to be packaged with scupulous care when being sent through the post; publishers will provide suitable guidance as to how to do this. Among the chief precautions you should take are: never write on the back of a photograph in anything other than pencil; separate photographs with sheets of paper; do not allow a paper clip (still less a staple!) to come into contact with the surface of an illustration or photograph; do not affix labels to the back of highly detailed photographs (the resulting change in contour can distort the reproduced image); draw symbols, cropping lines (i.e. lines indicating areas of the figure which are not to be reproduced) on an overlay, rather than directly onto the illustration.

Conclusion

This chapter has endeavoured to outline the principles which underlie the appropriate use of figures and tables. When used judiciously, graphics can do much to enhance your writing, in terms of both its intelligibility and its aesthetic appeal. However, like all communication techniques, figures and tables will only fulfil a useful purpose if they are constructed with care and used with discrimination. Unintelligible tables or figures which are poorly constructed, or made to have a visual impact at the cost of clarity, will only serve to confuse or even mislead the reader. An awareness of the strengths and weaknesses of various graphic forms will help to avoid such errors.

Chapter

9

Getting Published

Before you consider publishing your work it is as well to realize that publishing houses are commercial businesses whose aim is to make a profit. Kerton reminds us that:

> None will publish your book because they like you, because they see it as an act of charity, or because they think your words are so meaningful that it's only right and proper for the whole world to hear them. They will publish your book only if they feel sure enough people will buy it to make them a profit. (1986: 93)

It follows from this that your work must not only be of a high standard but must also be needed or desired by a fairly large number of people, especially if you are thinking of writing a book. This having been said, Cormack emphasizes that:

> Contrary to what some writers believe, editors are friendly people who try hard to enable and encourage professionals to develop their writing skills to the full, they have an obvious vested interest in stimulating the flow of high quality written material, it would not be in their interest to turn down good manuscripts out of hand or to discourage writers with potential. (1984: 5)

Where should you start?

Some people start their writing career by writing a book, but there can be no doubt that writing articles provides a valuable apprenticeship in which the confidence and skill to write a book may be gained. Writing articles also gives the writer credibility and visibility which can be so important when the first book is proposed. Writing articles will help you to build expertise in your chosen subject as well as improving your writing skills.

There is, of course, no need to write a full length book on your own. Many people prefer to write in collaboration with another or in teams. It may be that you cannot face a large amount of writing, that you need moral support, or that you lack expertise in certain areas. It is not even necessary for every team member to write, for example one may have carried out some interesting research which another agrees to write up. A further possibility is to edit a book. The rôle of the editor is to contact potential authors to write the various chapters, and to coordinate their contributions into a well-structured product. The editor usually contributes a few chapters as well, although this is not essential.

Market research

Before presenting either your ideas or your work to a journal editor or publisher, it is vital that you carry out some thorough market research. You should always write with a particular journal in mind and only present your ideas to a publisher who is likely to be interested in them. It is not a good idea to 'do the rounds' as it can waste a lot of time, and editors may get annoyed if they think you have not taken the trouble to look carefully at their publications before submitting your work. Many journal editors will provide you with a 'contributor's guide' which is valuable in giving you some idea of the kind of material they want.

Have a really good look at likely journals and magazines to see if your work would be appropriate. Note the length and content of articles, the length of sentences and paragraphs, and the complexity of the language. The typical reader can often be identified by the advertisements, the letters page and the illustrations. Find out which journals and magazines need freelance writers; you may choose to telephone the editors and ask, but much can be gleaned by studying the contents page. Always avoid subject areas covered by regular writers. With regard to books, browse around libraries and bookshops to check how many there are on your proposed subject. If you see a book in which the style and content appear to fit your ideas, or a series within which your work could fit, make a note of the publisher. It is usually pointless, however, to discuss your idea with a publisher who has recently published a book on precisely the same topic that you have in mind.

The Writers' and Artists' Yearbook and *The Writer's Handbook*, which are published every year, are very useful in identifying suitable journals and publishers. Publishers can also be approached for their catalogues. There is, however, no substitute for your own market research. If, having carried out the research, you find your idea or article is rejected by your chosen editor or publisher, do not hesitate to approach another.

Query letters

If you intend to write a book it is important to sell your idea and get a contract before you start writing. There is a very large market for non-fiction books; Linton (1988) points out that in 1986 there were 50,000 new non-fiction titles published in the United Kingdom. Non-fiction books can basically be divided into two types 'information books' and 'instruction books', although there is a great deal of overlap. It is much easier to publish non-fiction than fiction, but despite this, only one or two per cent of unsolicited manuscripts are accepted by publishers.

If you have a clear idea, enough material to write a book, and feel sufficiently confident to write it, then a suitable publisher should be approached; their business is publishing and they will be very pleased to hear from you. If you have written a number of articles and are recognized as being a specialist in a particular field, the publisher may contact you. You may also be approached by journal editors to write articles, especially if you have written for them before. Failing this, you should approach the publisher with a query letter; it gives a good impression if you address the person concerned by name. You need to state your proposed subject, your reasons for wanting to write the book, the proposed length of the book, at whom it is aimed, whether there are any competing books, and why you are the best person to write it. Say if you have had anything published already and offer to supply any titles with content similar to the book you are proposing. It is important to be concise and honest, but, nevertheless, you must sell yourself. Type the letter and enclose a stamped addressed envelope. Publishers and editors sometimes take rather a long time to reply because they need to seek advice and assess the viability of publishing and marketing your book, so be patient. If the publisher is interested you will be asked to write a synopsis and perhaps to supply one or two sample chapters.

With regard to articles, a query letter is not really necessary if the piece is short and does not involve you in too much work. A short business-like letter should simply be enclosed with the article and addressed to the editor by name. It is always good policy to enclose a stamped addressed envelope. A query letter is advisable, however, if the article is likely to involve a great deal of work, time or expense; it may be that the editor has a similar article in the pipeline. Remember that journal editors work about three months in advance, so if you want your article to be published by a specific date it should be sent in good time. If your writing pertains to a recent conference, however, the editor may be persuaded to squeeze your article in before the event is completely forgotten.

The synopsis

The synopsis is a brief account of what you intend to write. If the publisher's editor is interested in your idea you may be given verbal or written guidance on how to prepare the synopsis. It is written to enable the publisher to consider your ideas in greater depth and to provide suggestions and feed-back. Basically, a brief outline, of no more than a hundred words, is given for each chapter, as well as details of the readership for whom the book is intended, the purpose of the book and any existing books which are likely to compete with it. You will not be expected to adhere strictly to the synopsis when you start to write, it will merely serve as a guide.

Having presented your synopsis, you may be asked to meet the publisher's editor, perhaps over lunch, to discuss your ideas in greater depth. Publishing may seem to be shrouded in mystery at first, but do not be afraid to ask questions or to disagree. This having been said, it is important to listen to all the advice that is given; the editor wants you to succeed and the advice given is usually very valuable. Your proposal will be reviewed by one or two experts in the field; following this it may be provisionally accepted, rejected, or you may be asked to amend it in some way; it is usual to be asked to make some alterations. If it is provisionally accepted a publishing committee meeting will take place, comprising editorial, sales and marketing personnel. This will lead to the acceptance or the rejection of your proposal. If it is accepted you will be issued with a contract to prepare the work. If it is rejected you should certainly approach another publisher.

It is not a good idea to approach more than one publisher or journal editor with your ideas or work at the same time. It may be tempting to do so, but it gives a bad impression if you are accepted by both and then have to back away from one; remember you may want to approach that editor again one day. It may also have the effect of providing competitors with your ideas.

Rejections

All writers have their work rejected from time to time and it is important not to get discouraged or disheartened by this. Legat (1986) points out that John Braine sent the manuscript of his novel *Room at the Top* to thirty-eight publishers before it was accepted.

There are many reasons for rejection. It may be to do with the standard of your work; for example the title and first few lines may have failed to hold the editor's interest, the presentation may have been poor, it may have been the wrong length, or the structure may have been too loose, leading to confusion. However, rejections are just as likely to be due to factors unrelated to the quality of your writing; your work may, for example, fail to fit in with the publisher's current ideas, clash with a similar book or article which has already been accepted, or be considered unprofitable. Alternatively, your ideas may simply be too radical for the journal or publisher concerned. If you are told why your work or idea has been rejected listen carefully and learn from what is said, but do not hesitate to approach someone else.

Contracts

Before setting out to write a non-fiction book you should ensure that you have a contract. Publishers and contracts vary, but the contract you receive is usually a standard agreement, some of which can be amended; it should not be regarded as binding and inflexible until it is signed by both parties, but its clauses have usually stood the test of law and their wording, if agreed, is best left intact. Always read the contract carefully and if you do not understand any part of it, which is quite likely as it will be written in legal language, ask the editor for clarification. The Society of Authors and the Writers' Guild of Great Britain are organizations which work on behalf of writers and will give advice on contracts and other business matters. Authors can join these societies when their first full-length book has been accepted for publication. Contracts are not normally issued for the writing of articles, but you will be issued one if you contribute to an edited book.

The contract is a detailed statement laying out the obligations of both the writer and the publisher. It gives the provisional title of the book, its agreed length and the date of delivery of the manuscript. It is important not to be pressured into a date which is too early for you, and if you later discover, through unforeseen circumstances, that you cannot deliver the manuscript on time, do not panic, just give the publisher as much notice of the delay as possible. Remember, however, that your delay constitutes an infringement of the agreement and that the publisher is free to refuse the manuscript. If you want to write more than one book it is as well to keep on the right side of the publisher and to be reliable. It is always easier to have a second idea or piece of work accepted if the first was carried out in a professional manner.

The contract will also state the royalties you will receive – that is, the percentage of the publisher's receipts from sales of the book. It will also state when you will be paid. Royalties vary according to the type of book and its complexity, but usually range between 10 and 12.5 per cent of net receipts and are payable at agreed dates. If a manuscript is to be written within a tight schedule, some publishers may be prepared to pay an advance on the royalties when the book is in progress and again when it is first printed. The contract will also state the percentage of the payment you will receive if your work is translated or presented in a different medium, for example on the radio or television. These payments are referred to as subsidiary rights.

The contract usually gives the publisher the right to ask authors to amend their work and authors must agree not to write a book for another publisher which is likely to compete. It gives the date of publication, which is usually six months to a year after handing over the manuscript, and ensures that the publisher has full control of production – the printing, pricing, binding and cover design – although the writer's suggestions are always considered.

Writers must sign a declaration indicating that their work is not plagiarized or libellous or likely to attract other types of legal action. The writer agrees to read the proofs in a given period of time and, if the book does well, to revise it at a future date, or to allow someone else to do so. The contract may make it the writer's responsibility to pay for the cost of illustrations, the index and the proof corrections should they exceed a specified percentage of the original typesetting costs; such payments are usually paid by the publisher and deducted from the royalties. The writer may also be required to get permission to use other people's texts, diagrams and tables. The publisher usually agrees to supply the writer with a small number of books free on publication and a discount if more books are required. When the contract has been read and fully understood it should be signed and returned. In due course a copy signed by the publisher will be sent to the writer. (For details of the legal aspects of publishing, including the contract, the reader is referred to chapter 10.)

Agents

Some writers have agents to help them get work published on a regular basis. Agents concern themselves with the business side of writing, leaving the author free to write. They find new outlets for their clients, query contracts, and try to get the best possible deals. It is really only successful and regular writers who benefit from the services of agents. Approximately ten per cent of authors' profits are paid to them as commission, and, as they need to make a living, they are not interested in authors who do not write regularly or have not yet published a book.

Presentation

When you have revised your work as much as possible, care should be taken over the presentation. In a competitive market it is possible that your work will never be read if the presentation is poor. A professional attitude to your work will mean that editors are more likely to commission or accept your articles again. Your work should always be typed or printed with double line spacing on A4 paper with generous margins to allow the editor to write comments. Number the pages and always use a black typewriter or printer ribbon and a standard typeface. Indicate clearly where diagrams, pictures and tables should be placed in the text, number them carefully and place them at the back of the script. If you use a word processor, the editor may prefer your article or book-manuscript on disk, and may require more than one copy. Always keep a copy for yourself. Many publishers and editors provide guidelines concerning the layout of your work which, in the case of books, can be very specific, so you should ask for these and follow them carefully.

When writing a full-length book, errors will inevitably occur. The copy editor will help safeguard against these appearing in the finished book, but it is a mistake to rely on editors too heavily; the fact that they go over your writing is no excuse for your work to be shoddy. There is less likelihood of errors if you polish your work thoroughly and present it as neatly and clearly as you can; a few tidy alterations are acceptable. In the case of a full-length manuscript it is safer to send a copy by registered mail, or alternatively to hand it over to the editor in person. Always make sure to keep a copy.

The publishing process

Once the manuscript has been handed over to the publisher there is a short, and usually welcome, period of inactivity for the writer. During this period the editor will read the manuscript through and may send the whole of it, or a sample of chapters, to a few knowledgeable people, for example those who are involved in teaching the subject, for their comments and opinions. The writer may then be asked to make amendments. The manuscript will then be worked upon by the copy editor, who will tidy up any grammatical, punctuation and spelling errors and make sure that everything is clearly expressed and appears accurate. The copy editor will also make changes, not because things are necessarily wrong, but because every publisher has its own particular house style which dictates the ways in which the work is presented, for example whether numbers should be written out, which spelling to use if there is more than one alternative and the referencing system. Writers are usually given a booklet in advance so that they can follow the publisher's house style as far as possible.

In due course the writer will receive the copy editor's comments and will be asked to clarify various points and make corrections. If earlier work was done well this should not be a major job. The copy editor's comments are usually very helpful and should be welcomed by writers as they are likely to improve the standard of the book, but you should not be afraid to disagree with them or ask for clarification. There will then be a further period of inactivity for the writer during which time the manuscript will be printed into a long, continuous text known as the galley proofs. These are checked for accuracy by the writer and the copy editor. The corrected proofs are then printed in pages and if the book contains illustrations these are placed in the text. The page proofs resemble the actual book and are sent to the author to check. They are also checked by the editorial staff. The author will also be asked to check for accuracy any illustrations that have been prepared. (For further information on illustrations and photographs the reader is referred to chapter 8.)

Proof reading is an important task and should be carried out meticulously. Each word must be inspected in an attempt to remove every error. No new matter should be inserted at this stage without discussion with the publisher; if there has been a major change, for example a new Act of Parliament, alterations may be essential. There is a standard way of correcting proofs where specific symbols are used; the system is not difficult and you will learn it very quickly. A list of the symbols appears in BSI (British Standards Institution) Standard BS 5261. Complete copies of the Standard can be obtained from: BSI Publications, Linford Wood, Milton Keynes, Buckinghamshire MK14 6LE, UK. If you send an article to a professional journal, proofs will also be sent to you for correction. At about this time the cover of the book will be designed, and the 'blurb' on the back cover written by one of the editors. The opinion of the writer may or may not be sought. The book will usually be published about eight weeks after the page proofs are returned to the publisher.

The number of copies printed in the first instance varies. Complimentary copies will be sent to influential people and to journal editors for review. You may be involved in promotional activities to sell the book, such as attendance at a launch. Another way of increasing sales is to write a journal article on the same subject, mentioning that the book is about to be published. If the book sells well and more copies are required, it will be reprinted and there is a further opportunity to correct any typographical errors that remain and to make minor alterations. It is a good idea to keep a list of any errors you see.

If the book is still selling successfully after a few years you may be asked to revise it, to prepare a second edition. The material must all be updated and new chapters may be added; it is usually a major piece of work. If, on the other hand, the book does not sell very well it will go out of print or, if existing copies remain unsold, they may be sold off very cheaply, a process known as 'remaindering'. You will normally be given the option of buying the copies yourself. Publishers are skilful at gauging likely sales so this situation does not arise very often, but predicting sales is always something of a guessing game.

Vanity publishing and self-publishing

With vanity publishing writers make a financial contribution to publishing their own books and are largely responsible for selling them. The usual advice is 'don't do it'. Kerton (1986) believes that the only test of a good book is whether or not an established publisher will publish it.

Self-publishing is practised when the author takes on the entire responsibility for the production of the book. It requires money, a head for business, a very reliable and experienced printer, and the confidence that the book will sell well and not make a loss. Hines (1990) believes that it should be reserved for books with an assured market, in which case it may be more profitablee for the author than conventional publishing. It may also be the only way of getting a minority interest book published. Despite this the usual advice is still 'don't do it'. (For examples of these and other non-conventional publishing methods, readers are referred to Hines, 1990.)

Publishing articles

Selling and publishing articles is simpler than selling and publishing books, although equal care must be taken by the writer. In the case of the 'light-weight' specialist newspapers all you need to do is to send your article to the editor who will make a decision about whether or not to accept it. It should be accompanied by a covering letter. If it is accepted you will be informed and it will appear in the newspaper a few weeks or months later. It is not usually worth writing a query letter unless you are thinking of producing a long article or a series of articles. One of the authors (SF) wrote a series of four articles on teaching methods in 1989, without writing a query letter, and they were rejected. The articles totalled 10,000 words and had involved a considerable amount of work. Fortunately they were accepted by another publication, but it could have meant a lot of wasted effort. With light-weight newspapers you will not receive any proofs to correct and your article may be changed by the editorial staff. With professional and academic journals, proofs are supplied and changes are only made with the writer's permission.

When you submit your article to a professional journal it will be sent to several experts, usually from the profession concerned, for their comments; the process is termed 'peer review'. These people help the editor to decide whether your article should be accepted, accepted with modifications, or rejected. If it is accepted with modifications there is usually some room for negotiation. This all takes considerable time and it is not unusual to wait for six months or more before seeing your article in print, or receiving the payment, if any.

The financial rewards of writing articles vary enormously. The top price expected for writing in a leading national newspaper may be as high as £200 for 1,000 words. In journals and magazines it varies widely, with many paying nothing at all. Editors may pay differential rates according to the writer's skill and status, and it may therefore be worth entering into negotiations for the best possible deal, especially when you are established. Although the financial rewards of writing are generally not that great, it can lead to other fairly lucrative opportunities such as running workshops and free-lance teaching. (For further detail of the whole of the publishing process the reader is referred to Legat, 1991.)

Conclusion

Spender (1981) points out that, in a very fundamental way, ideas and research findings which are not in print do not exist. If you have completed a research project, no matter how small, or if you have some interesting ideas or experiences which may help or be of interest to others, try to publish them or your work and expertise will remain unknown by all but a few.

10

Writing and the Law

This chapter will explore some of the legal issues concerned with writing. As such, it will not endeavour to offer a fully comprehensive account of copyright, defamation and allied issues. There are specialist legal texts available which deal with these topics, and specific legal advice should be sought from a professional lawyer. Instead, certain aspects of the law will be covered in fairly general terms, so as to alert the intending author to some of the legal pitfalls and obstacles that may be encountered. Some of the legal rights which a writer possesses in respect of his or her work will also be considered.

The law discussed will apply to England and Wales and sometimes – especially in the case of copyright law – to Scotland and Northern Ireland. General principles, however, will often apply, to a greater or lesser degree, to other countries.

Contracts

The contract between writer and publisher was addressed in general terms in chapter 9; the specifically legal implications of the contract will be considered here.

A contract is a legally binding agreement between two or more parties. It contains a number of terms, and if one or more of these are breached, the responsible party is liable to a civil action for damages from the other party. A serious breach of a term may result in the termination of the contract.

The terms usually contained in a publishing contract were examined in chapter 9. Of these, perhaps the most important from the writer's point of view (and probably from the publisher's point of view also) is the timescale agreed in the contract for completion of the work. The contract will usually specify the date by which the completed manuscript should be delivered, in its entirety and in an acceptable form, to the publisher. Publishers are fully aware of the fact that unforeseen circumstances may make it harder than was anticipated to meet deadlines, and that authors may experience other unexpected difficulties in the process of producing the finished manuscript. Consequently, they will normally try to be as flexible as is reasonably possible with regard to these contractual terms. In most cases, publishers will consider requests for extensions of deadlines sympathetically, especially if they are negotiated well in advance of the original delivery date. After all, it is hardly in their interests to publish a hurriedly-completed manuscript. However, it is as well to be aware of the possible outcome if such accommodation between the parties cannot be arrived at. Should you, as the author, fail to meet the delivery date when it is 'of the essence' in the contract, the publisher may decline to proceed with the work, and you may even be sued for damages, in particular for any financial loss which the publishing house may incur as a result of the late delivery (or indeed the non-delivery) of the manuscript. If it can be shown that the manuscript has been completed, the publisher may be able to obtain a court order requiring you to hand it over. It must be emphasized, however, that these are the worst eventualities, and can be prevented or circumvented by an open and cooperative relationship between writer and publisher.

Another important contractual term which is usually to be found in publishing agreements is an indemnity given to the publisher by the author in the event of a successful action for libel, blasphemy, breach of copyright, or similar legal action, occasioned by material in the book. In this respect, it is particularly important to ensure that any treatment recommendations, such as prescribed exercises, treatment dosages and stated contraindications, are accurate and in keeping with acceptable professional practice. A similar degree of care is required with regard to breach of copyright, and it is to this subject that we will now turn.

Copyright

Copyright is part of intellectual property law, the section of the law that also governs patents, designs and similar creative works. As such, it affords legal rights to the author. The following quotation describes the scope of copyright:

> Copyright protection subsists in original works of authorship fixed in any tangible medium of expression, now known or later developed, from which they can be perceived, reproduced, or otherwise communicated, either directly or with the aid of a machine or device. (Nolan and Nolan-Haley, 1990: 336)

The legislative source of copyright law is the Copyright, Designs and Patents Act 1988; the copyright provisions of the Act came into force on 1 August 1989. There is no international copyright law as such, but some degree of protection is afforded by the Berne Convention (1886) and the Universal Copyright Convention (1952), both of which have been revised and extended since their creation (Flint, 1990). Most countries are signatories to one or both of these conventions, China being a notable exception. The significance of the conventions is that their signatories undertake to provide reciprocal copyright protection to works of each other's nationals, and declare that the protection so provided will conform to certain minimum standards. In order to secure such reciprocal protection you, as copyright owner, should include in your work the copyright symbol, ©, followed by your name and the year of first publication anywhere in the world; this is especially important in order to secure protection in countries which are not signatories to the Berne Convention but which are members of the Universal Copyright Convention, such as the countries making up the former Union of Soviet Socialist Republics (Flint, 1990).

The details of copyright

It is important to state what can be subject to copyright, so as to dispel any misconceptions as to its precise nature and scope. There is one category of works in the Copyright, Designs and Patents Act 1988 that is particularly relevant to writers. This is the category comprising 'original literary, dramatic, musical or artistic works'. A 'literary work' is any work which is written, spoken or sung in recorded form. It includes tables, or other compilations, and computer programs. 'Artistic work' is widely defined in the 1988 Act, and includes photographs. Such works will embrace virtually everything a therapist is likely to produce as an author.

It is, however, important to appreciate that there is no copyright on ideas, only on their expression in a material form (sometimes referred to as 'fixation'). As Phillips and Firth (1990: 115–116) point out:

> You can have enough lofty ideas to fill a think-tank and yet find that you have not produced an original 'work' until you have given those ideas an appropriate form. Literary works may be written, spoken or sung to a tune, but copyright cannot subsist until the literary work is recorded, in writing or otherwise.

Copyright protection takes effect from the creation of a work, even if it is not subsequently published or otherwise reproduced. Thus a dissertation, a report, or teaching materials for an individual's sole purposes are protected in the same way as a book or other publication which is reproduced. Note, however, that the 1988 Act provides that, subject to the terms of a contract (e.g. of employment), the copyright in literary works produced by employees in the course of their work belongs to the employer. Nor does a work need to be specially registered in order to enjoy copyright protection, because copyright is acquired automatically when the work is recorded. The 1988 Act has no registration requirements for copyright.

Copyright has a 'lifetime'; it generally expires fifty years after the end of the calendar year of the author's death. In the case of jointly-authored works, copyright extends for a similar period from the death of the author who dies last (unless, of course, the authors' contributions to the work are distinguishable and separately copyrighted).

The ownership of copyright is unrelated to ownership of the material in or upon which the literary or artistic work is published. Thus Cornish (1989) points out that although the sender of a letter implicitly transfers ownership of the letter to its recipient, he or she does not thereby transfer the copyright in its contents. In a similar way, you as a writer may own a manuscript, but have no right to publish it as the copyright in its contents may be held by another, e.g. a publishing house. Nonetheless, the copyright of any work is the author's unless and until it is contractually agreed otherwise, and thus the contract between writer and publisher usually makes some provision for the transfer of copyright from author to publisher.

Finally, a work must be original in order to enjoy copyright protection. This does not mean that it must contain 'new' material, or material which embodies a certain level of creativity or inventiveness. Rather, '[o]riginality in the copyright sense simply means that there is a direct causative link between the author's mental conception and the work which emanates from his hand' (Phillips and Firth, 1990: 117). The crucial factor, therefore, is that the work in question *originates* from the author, rather than from somebody else.

Exceptions to copyright

There are a number of 'permitted acts' which do not infringe copyright, and these are provided for in the 1988 Act. Those of most relevance to the author are found in the provisions relating to 'fair dealing'. Thus, 'fair dealing' with a literary, dramatic, musical or artistic work for the purposes of research or private study does not infringe any copyright in the work. Likewise, 'fair dealing' with a work for the purposes of criticism or review – of that or another work – does not infringe copyright, provided that it is accompanied by sufficient acknowledgment.

Plagiarism

Plagiarism is a term which describes:

> The act of appropriating the literary composition of another, or parts or passages of his writings, or the ideas or language of the same, and passing them off as the product of one's own mind. If the material is protected by copyright, such act may constitute an offense of copyright infringement. (Nolan and Nolan-Haley, 1990: 1150)

As this quotation indicates, plagiarism includes any unauthorized appropriation of the ideas of another, legally or illegally. Plagiarism of another's ideas is not necessarily breach of copyright, for, as noted earlier, copyright exists not in ideas themselves, but in their expression. The student who passes off another's work as his or her own is a plagiarist and, even if copyright is infringed, is unlikely to face legal action; nonetheless the student may face severe penalties from the educational institution to whom the work is submitted. On the other hand, the 'professional' author who does likewise may, in certain circumstances, be sued for damages, and even prosecuted for breach of copyright. In either case, an accusation of plagiarism is an extremely unpleasant experience, and may irreparably tarnish your professional reputation.

Plagiarism is, in any case, far easier to detect than is generally supposed. Writers readily recognize their own work, even if it is craftily adapted, and tutors soon become adept at identifying unattributed paraphrases or similar 'borrowings' in student coursework.

Avoiding plagiarism which amounts to breach of copyright

How, then, should you avoid an accusation of plagiarism involving breach of copyright in respect of what you have written? There are several safeguards which should be followed. The first is to ensure that any quotations are indicated as such, by the use of quotation marks and/or separation from the main text of your work, and that due reference is made to their source (see chapter 6). In this way, you make it clear that the material in question is not being passed off as your own. Note, however, that if you intend to use an extract or quotation which is 'substantial', you may require the express permission of the copyright holder; merely acknowledging its source may be insufficient. In addition, you may be required to pay a fee. Unfortunately, there is no clear, agreed definition of what constitutes a 'substantial' part of another writer's work. What is clear, however, is that the word 'substantial' applies both qualitatively as well as quantitatively. Thus, Flint (1990: 60) states:

> If the most vital part of a work is copied – even though it may not be a very large part of a work – it will nevertheless be considered to be a substantial part for the purpose of deciding whether or not there is an infringement [of copyright].

Note that the contract between publisher and author usually stipulates that the responsibility for obtaining any necessary permissions to reproduce copyright material lies with the author.

A second safeguard is to be aware that an act of copying does not need to be verbatim to constitute a breach of copyright. Legat points out that '[y]ou can't get away with changing the words if you still use the same sentence structure, and the same kind of paragraphing, and all the same facts' (Legat, 1991: 211). Consider, for example, the following extract from a recent book on hearing-impairment in children:

> When a manually coded English system is selected as the initial method of exposing a child to language, it is critical that the family become fluent as rapidly as possible in the combination of signs and speech. Care must be taken that the child's family and educational personnel are trained in the signs that are peculiar to the selected system. Obviously, serious problems will arise if different symbols are used in different settings. (Maxon and Brackett, 1992: 47)

This could be paraphrased in such a way that very little of the original specific phraseology remains:

If a decision is made to adopt a manually coded English system as the primary method of introducing a child to language, it is imperative for the child's family to achieve fluency in the combination of signs and speech that constitute the system in the shortest possible time. Within the chosen language system, assiduous training should be provided for the family, and also for those with whom the child will come into contact in the educational setting, in the relevant signs. If there is a mismatch between symbols used in different contexts, this is clearly undesirable.

However, there are unmistakable signs that the second extract is based on the first. The same points are made in the same order, and in the same number of sentences. Each unit of sense in the original can readily be matched with its counterpart in the 'copy'. Moreover, the emphasis within the description given is virtually identical ('it is critical'/'it is imperative'; 'obviously'/'clearly'). Plagiarism has clearly occurred here, and if such copying can be shown to be 'substantial' in terms of the 1988 Act, a successful action for breach of copyright could be brought.

Even the fact that you have used substantially the same references or other source material may give rise to a charge of plagiarism, however dissimilar your textual treatment of the topic. It must be said, however, that such an accusation would usually be very difficult to substantiate, as writers dealing with the same subject are in many cases almost bound to utilize much the same corpus of existing literature.

This leads us to the third safeguard. If you do find a passage in another's work on which you decide to base your own treatment of the topic in question, acknowledge the fact that you have done so by means of more than a simple reference. You could, for example, introduce a footnote at the appropriate point along the following lines: 'The section that follows is indebted to Haynes's discussion of this issue (Haynes, 1987 chap 6)'. Alternatively, within the main text you could lead into your discussion in a manner such as this: 'Attention will now be focused on [a certain topic], and here I will draw upon the discussion to be found in Haynes (1987 chap 6)'. Bear in mind that under the 1988 Act there must be 'sufficient acknowledgment' of any material quoted, and while a simple bibliographic reference may often fulfil this requirement, in some instances a fuller acknowledgment, such as those illustrated above, may be prudent.

The final safeguard you should take is simply that of consulting an appropriate authority in any cases of doubt. Your publisher will have considerable experience of matters to do with copyright, and advice can also be sought from the Society of Authors or the Writers' Guild of Great Britain (see chapter 9). In particularly difficult cases, the services of a lawyer specializing in intellectual property law may be required. It should be noted, however, that poor legal advice is no defence to a breach of copyright (though if such advice is given the legal adviser may, in certain circumstances, be sued for the tort of negligent misstatement). From a practical point of view, insurance can be sought for 'protection' against successful civil suits for breach of copyright.

Quite apart from the legal implications of plagiarism, to appropriate the fruits of somebody else's labour is, at best, disrespectful.

How to determine who owns the copyright

The author of a literary, dramatic, musical or artistic work is the person who creates it; this person may or may not be the copyright owner. It is usually relatively easy to determine the copyright owner of a written work. In books, this is generally indicated on the back of the title page by means of the copyright symbol. Books are generally copyright as a whole, though in the case of multi-authored or edited books the copyright of different chapters may be attributed to individual authors. In journals, copyright is customarily indicated at the top or the bottom of the first page of each article. Very often, the copyright will be owned by the publisher rather than by an individual writer, and in such cases it is of course from the publisher that permission to use material should be sought. However, it is also a matter of courtesy to inform the author (in the case of a book) or the editor (in the case of a journal) that you intend using the material in question, and that the appropriate permission has been (or is being) obtained from the publisher. If the copyright ownership of the work is not obvious, do not assume you can immediately go ahead and make free use of the material; the law will require you to have made reasonable efforts to discover the identity of the copyright owner.

Quoting unpublished work

There may be occasions when you wish to quote from unpublished material, such as a thesis or dissertation, a report with a restricted circulation, or the proceedings of a meeting or conference which have not been made publicly available. Here, you should seek the permission of the original author before doing so. This is not only for legal reasons connected with the copyright of the material (recall that works do not have to be published to enjoy copyright protection), but also out of courtesy. By publishing a written work, the author has committed it expressly to public scrutiny, and has implicitly declared an intention to 'stand by' what he or she has said. It usually represents the writer's fully-developed view on the subject in question. However, in the case of unpublished material, such as in the examples above, the author may have been discussing 'work in progress', exploring a tentative theory, or advancing preliminary ideas on a certain topic. You should therefore check that the source you wish to quote from represents a standpoint with which the author would still wish to be associated, and that he or she is happy to be publicly identified with it.

Protecting your own copyright work

If you own the copyright of published written work and you detect unauthorized or unattributed use of your writing which amounts to breach of copyright, the law affords you a number of remedies; you can seek an injunction to prevent further use of the material, obtain damages for any loss you may have incurred, and even, in some circumstances, seize the offending material yourself (though the last of these is not recommended to any reader with a less than thorough understanding of the relevant law!). Before taking any steps you should take advice from your publisher, from an association such as the Society of Authors or from a lawyer. What you should not do is bandy about charges of plagiarism, especially in any public medium, for should your accusations prove groundless, you could then find yourself being sued for defamation.

If, on the other hand, the copyright to the work is held by a publishing house, you should simply inform your publisher, who will initiate the necessary steps.

Confidentiality

It is important to respect the privacy of any individuals whom you may identify in your writing. In patients' notes, it is of course vitally important to make it clear whom you are writing about. However, when writing case reports and similar documents for use outside the immediate clinical situation (e.g. in a case study for publication or as part of student coursework), there is no reason to identify a patient by name. To do so is a breach of confidentiality and, while this may not in itself be legally actionable, any consequent loss incurred by the patient could be recovered from you in a civil action. Moreover, breach of confidentiality may be contrary to the terms of a contract of employment. The use of illustrations requires special care: Brazier reports the sobering case of a young man who received treatment in hospital, only to discover in a medical textbook, some time later, a full-face, full-frontal picture of himself naked (Brazier, 1992). If you publish photographs of patients, you should ensure that you have their consent to do so, and, unless they agree otherwise, that steps are taken to conceal their identity, such as by blanking out their eyes. Most publishers will insist on this.

Defamation

Defamatory statements are those which 'discredit or lower the plaintiff in the estimation of right thinking members of society' (Harlow, 1987: 107). This may occur through the spoken word (in which case it is referred to as slander) or in print or a television or radio transmission (when it is known as libel). If defamation can be shown to have occurred, damages may be awarded, so as to compensate the plaintiff for the injury done to his or her reputation. In addition, libel is actionable in itself, and in some cases of slander, proof of specific damage may not be required.

It is important to note that a plaintiff need not establish an *intention* to libel on the part of the author: the significant factor is how the relevant statements will be understood by the public, and any explicit or implicit defamatory inferences that are likely to be drawn from them.

Needless to say, therapists are in much less danger of libelling an individual in their professional writing than, say, a journalist or a political commentator. There are, however, a few instances in which special care should be taken to avoid a possible action for libel:

(1) Beware of denigrating the professional competence or standing of another practitioner. Parsons (1993) notes that a statement can be defamatory 'even if it does no more than contain an attack on a person's professional integrity or a criticism of the way he or she carries out a job'. In particular, do not refer to somebody as 'unqualified' just because you do not recognize the status of his or her training; the fact that a practitioner does not have the qualifications required for state registration is not to say that the individual is 'unqualified'.

(2) If reviewing the work of another – in a book review, for example – ensure that any criticisms you make are objective. This is not to say that you cannot express a personal opinion, but to emphasize that your views should not appear to be motivated by personal animus. Your criticisms should be directed at the work, not at its author.

(3) In view of patients' increasing access to their notes (see below), it is important to be objective and non-judgemental when writing about patients or clients, and to avoid committing anything to paper which might be construed as defamatory.

Clinical writing

Since November 1987, the Data Protection Act of 1984 has afforded patients in the United Kingdom a right of access, in certain circumstances, to any health records held in a computerized form, and under the Access to Medical Reports Act 1988 patients have a similar right in respect of medical reports drawn up in relation to employment or insurance cover, whether such reports are computerized or not (Dimond, 1990). The Access to Health Records Act 1990 has extended patients' rights in this area, allowing them to apply, in certain circumstances, for access to any manually held health records compiled after November 1991, both in the National Health Service and in the private sector (Brazier, 1992). Specific regulations cover which individuals are entitled to have access to such records and in what form these will be presented. Furthermore, some health authorities are now granting patients routine access to general medical and nursing records, even without any formal request. The significance of patient access to health records goes beyond the simple satisfaction of personal curiosity; it allows the rectification of omissions or inaccuracies.

These developments underline the need to ensure that clinical records are kept up-to-date and complete, and constructed with due circumspection. Should you find yourself in the unhappy position of being sued for professional negligence, your case notes may be admissible evidence. There are a few specific points that should be borne in mind. Each entry in the patient's notes should be signed and dated, and should be as contemporaneous as possible with the events to which it refers. It is vital to make full notes on any untoward incident that may have occurred during the care or treatment of a patient. Do not, however, explicitly attribute such incidents to professional incompetence or inefficiency (e.g. 'the patient's gait is poor due to misalignment of the prosthetic knee', 'the patient cannot adjust to his amputation as a result of inadequate pre-operative preparation'). Always make a note of the fact that a patient has consented to treatment, especially if it is of a potentially hazardous nature, and record all diagnostic tests, whether positive or negative.

Never obliterate an entry with a correction fluid such as Liquid Paper or Tippex, as this may suggest some form of tampering or concealment; rather, cross through anything to be deleted in such a way that the original is still legible. Copies should also be kept of all reports, such as summaries of home visits or letters to patients' general practitioners. Finally, student therapists are often well advised to have certain entries – especially those which may have potential legal implications – countersigned by a qualified member of staff.

Conclusion

This chapter has touched upon some of the legal issues which may confront the author. Therapists will be aware from their own experience in health care that society is becoming generally more aware of its rights and increasingly litigious, and this tendency is doubtless mirrored in respect of the written word. A general awareness of the likely legal pitfalls facing the writer – whether in relation to publishing or in everyday clinical practice – is therefore of timely importance. It must, however, be emphasized once more that what has been said in this chapter has been phrased in general terms and is not a substitute for obtaining qualified legal advice should the need arise.

References

Ahmad B. (1990) *Black Perspectives on Social Work*, Birmingham, Venture Press

Anderson J., Durston B. H., Poole M. (1970) *Thesis and Assignment Writing*, Sydney, John Wiley

ANSI (1969) *American National Standard for the Abbreviation of Titles of Periodicals*, New York, American National Standards Institute

Arnell P. (1985) Awareness of and access to physiotherapy-related publications: a professional necessity. *Physiotherapy* 71, 271

Ashburn A. (1982) A motor assessment for stroke patients. *Physiotherapy* 68, 109–113

Babbie E. (1989) *The Practice of Social Research*, 5th edn. Belmont, Wadsworth Publishing

Barrass R. (1982) *Students Must Write: a Guide to Better Writing in Course Work and Examinations*, London, Methuen

Barrass R. (1984) *Study! A Guide to Effective Study, Revision and Examination Techniques*, London, Chapman and Hall

Baxter C. (1988) *The Black Nurse: an Endangered Species*, Cambridge, National Extension College for Training in Health and Race

Baxter C., Poonia K., Ward L. et al. (1990) *Double Discrimination: Issues and Services for People with Learning Difficulties from Black and Ethnic Minority Communities*, London, King's Fund Centre/Commission for Racial Equality

Becker H. S. (1986) *Writing for Social Scientists*, Chicago, University of Chicago Press

Bohannon R. W. (1987) Core journals of physiotherapy. *Physiotherapy Practice* 3, 126–128

Bohannon R. W. (1988) How to find relevant references for a publication. *Physiotherapy Practice* 4, 41–44

Bohannon R. W., Gibson D. F. (1986) Citation analysis of physical therapy. A special communication. *Physical Therapy* 66, 540–541

Brazier M. (1992) *Medicine, Patients and the Law*, 2nd edn., Harmondsworth, Penguin

Brown G., Atkins M. (1988) *Effective Teaching in Higher Education*, London, Methuen

Brown R. A., Beck J. S. (1990) *Medical Statistics on Microcomputers*, London, British Medical Journal

BSI (1976) *Recommendations for Bibliographic References*, London, British Standards Institution

Butler R. N. (1975) *Why Survive? Being Old in America*, New York, Harper and Row

Buzan T. (1989) *Use Your Head*, 3rd edn., London, BBC Books

Chapman M., Mahon B. (1986) *Plain Figures*, London, HMSO

Cormack D. F. S. (1984) *Writing for Nursing and Allied Professions*, Oxford, Blackwell Scientific Publications

Cornish W. R. (1989) *Intellectual Property: Patents, Copyright, Trade Marks and Allied Rights*, London, Sweet & Maxwell

Currier D. P. (1975) Let's reduce the communication gap: how to present data in figures and tables. *Physical Therapy* 55, 768–772

Day R. A. (1989) *How to Write and Publish a Scientific Paper*, 3rd edn., Cambridge, Cambridge University Press

Dean E. (1986) Measuring professional eminence in physical therapy. *Physiotherapy Canada* 38, 4–5

DeLacey G., Record C., Wade J. (1985) How accurate are quotations and references in medical journals? *British Medical Journal* 291, 884–886

Dickersin K., Hewitt P. (1986) Look before you quote. *British Medical Journal* 293, 1000–1002

Dimond B. (1990) *Legal Aspects of Nursing*, New York, Prentice Hall

Dixon B. R., Bouma G. D., Atkinson G. B. J. (1987) *A Handbook of Social Science Research*, Oxford, Oxford University Press

Dudley H. (1977) *The Presentation of Original Work in Medicine and Biology*, Edinburgh, Churchill Livingstone

Dunleavy P. (1986) *Studying for a Degree in the Humanities and Social Sciences*, London, Macmillan

Ehrlich, E., Flexner S. B., Carruth G., Hawkins J. M. (1980) *Oxford American Dictionary*, New York, Oxford University Press

Elbow P. (1981) *Writing with Power*, Oxford, Oxford University Press

Enrick N. L. (1972) *Effective Graphic Communication*, Princeton, Auerbach Publishers

Fletcher R. H. (1974) Auditing problem orientated medical records. A controlled experiment of speed, accuracy and identification of errors in medical care. *New England Journal of Medicine* 78, 751–762

Flint M. F. (1990) *A User's Guide to Copyright*, 3rd edn., London, Butterworths

French S. (1991) Setting a record straight. *Therapy Weekly* 18, 4

French S. (1992) Clinical interviewing. In *Physiotherapy: a Psychosocial Approach*, (ed. French S.), Oxford, Butterworth-Heinemann

Garton A., Pratt C. (1989) *Learning to be Literate – the Development of Spoken and Written Language*, Oxford, Basil Blackwell

Gordon P., Rosenberg D. (1989) *Daily Racism: the Press and Black People in Britain*, London, Runnymede Trust

Harlow C. (1987) *Understanding Tort Law*, London, Fontana Press

Harris P. (1986) *Designing and Reporting Experiments*, Milton Keynes, Open University Press

Hart H. (1983) *Hart's Rules for Compositors and Readers at the University Press Oxford*, 39th edn., Oxford, Oxford University Press

Hawthorne J. (1989) *30 Ways to Make Money in Writing*, London, Rosters

Hemphill B. J. (1982) *Evaluative Process in Psychiatric Occupational Therapy*, Thorofare, Charles B. Slack

Hicks C. M. (1988) *Practical Research Methods for Physiotherapists*, Edinburgh, Churchill Livingstone

Hill A. B., Hill I. D. (1991) *Bradford Hill's Principles of Medical Statistics*, 12th edn, London, Edward Arnold

Hines J. (1987) *The Way to Write Magazine Articles*, London, Elm Tree Books

Hines J. (1990) *The Way to Write Non-Fiction*, London, Elm Tree Books

Holmes N. (1984) *Designer's Guide to Creating Charts and Diagrams*, New York, Watson-Guptill

Huff D. (1973) *How to Lie with Statistics*, Harmondsworth, Penguin

ICMJE (1982) Uniform requirements for manuscripts submitted to biomedical journals: International Committee of Medical Journal Editors. *British Medical Journal* 284, 1766–1770

Kerlinger, F. N. (1973) *Foundations of Behavioral Research*, 2nd edn., New York, Holt, Rinehart and Winston

Kerton P. (1986) *The Freelance Writer's Handbook*, London, Ebury Press

Kidder L. H., Judd C. M. (1986) *Research Methods in Social*

Relations, 5th edn., New York, CBS College Publishing

Kirby M. (1981) To refer or not to refer. *Physiotherapy* 67, 50

Knowles R. (1987) Who's a pretty girl then? *Nursing Times* 23 (8th July), 58–59

Kolin P. C., Kolin J. L. (1980) *Professional Writing for Nurses in Education, Practice, and Research*, St Louis, C. V. Mosby

Leach C. (1988) Guidelines for data presentation. In *The Psychologist's Companion: a Guide to Scientific Writing for Students and Researchers*, (ed. Sternberg R. J.), Cambridge, Cambridge University Press

Legat M. (1986) *Writing for Pleasure and Profit*, London, Robert Hale

Legat M. (1991) *An Author's Guide 'to Publishing*, 2nd edn., London, Robert Hale

Lewis R. (1979) *How to Write Essays*, London, Heinemann

Ley P. (1988) *Communicating with Patients: Improving Communication, Satisfaction and Compliance*, London, Chapman and Hall

Linton I. (1988) *Writing for a Living*, London, Kogan Page

Lister M. (1989) Writing manuscripts for a scientific journal. *Physiotherapy Practice* 5, 147–155

Lobo H., Taylor C. (1988) *Hysterectomy and Vaginal Repair*, booklet for patients, Mayday Hospital, Thornton Heath

Lock S. (1982) Authors of the world unite. *British Medical Journal* 284, 1726–1727

Lyne P. A. (1989) Peer review of papers submitted for publication. *Physiotherapy Practice* 5, 17–23

McIlroy, J. (1990) Examinations. In *Making the Grade. Volume 2: Thinking and Writing*, (eds Jones B. and Johnson R.), Manchester, Manchester University Press

Marsh C. (1988) *Exploring Data: an Introduction to Data Analysis for Social Scientists*, Cambridge, Polity Press

Maxon A. B., Bracket D. (1992) *The Hearing-Impaired Child: Infancy through High School Years*, Boston, Andover Medical Publishers

Melzack R., Wall P. D. (1965) Pain mechanisms: a new theory. *Science* 150, 971–979

Miller C., Swift K. (1989) *The Handbook of Non-Sexist Writing for Writers, Editors and Speakers*, 2nd edn., London, The Women's Press

Newble D., Cannon R. (1990) *A Handbook for Teachers in Universities and Colleges*, London, Kegan Paul

Nolan J. R., Nolan-Haley J. M. (1990) *Black's Law Dictionary*, 6th edn., St Paul, West Publishing Co.

O'Connor M. (1978) Standardisation of bibliographical reference systems. *British Medical Journal* 1, 31–32

O'Connor M., Woodford F. P. (1978) *Writing Scientific Papers in English: an ELSE Ciba Foundation Guide for Authors*, London, Pitman Medical

Parsons D. (1993) The dangers of libel and how to avoid them. *British Medical Journal* 306, 253–255

Petrie J. C., McIntyre M. (1979) *The Problem Orientated Medical Record*, Edinburgh, Churchill Livingstone

Phillips J., Firth A. (1990) *Introduction to Intellectual Property Law*, 2nd edn., London, Butterworths

Poyer R. K. (1979) Inaccurate references in significant journals of science. *Bulletin of the Medical Library Association* 67, 396–398

Pritchard J. (1992) *Abuse of Elderly People: a Handbook for Professionals*, London, Jessica Kingsley

Reid N. G., Boore J. R. P. (1987) *Research Methods and Statistics in Health Care*, London, Edward Arnold

Roberts D. (1986) CATS: a new information service in physiotherapy. *Physiotherapy* 72, 533–535

Rowntree D. (1988) *Learn How to Study*, 3rd edn., London, Sphere Books

Schmid C. F., Schmid S. E. (1979) *Handbook of Graphic Presentation*, 2nd edn., New York, Ronald Press

Scholey M. E. (1985) Documentation: a means of professional development. *Physiotherapy* 71, 276–278

Shearer B. S., Wall J. C., Burnham J. F. (1992) Anatomy of a literature search. *Clinical Management* 12, 23–31

Shipman M. (1988) *The Limitations of Social Research*, 3rd edn., London, Longman

Sim J. (1986) Informed consent: ethical implications for physiotherapy. *Physiotherapy* 72, 584–587

Sim J. (1989) Methodology and morality in physiotherapy research. *Physiotherapy* 75, 237–243

Sim J. (1993) Communication, counselling and health education. In *Physiotherapy for Respiratory and Cardiac Problems*, (eds Webber B. A., Pryor J.), Edinburgh, Churchill Livingstone

Smith R. (1988) Problems with peer review and alternatives. *British Medical Journal* 296, 774–777

Spender D. (1981) The gatekeepers: a feminist critique of academic publishing. In *Doing Feminist Research* (ed. Roberts H.), London, Routledge & Kegan Paul

Spender D. (1985) *Man Made Language*, 2nd edn., London, Routledge & Kegan Paul

Sternberg R. J. (1988) *The Psychologist's Companion: a Guide to Scientific Writing for Students and Researchers*, Cambridge, Cambridge University Press

Tufte E. R. (1983) *The Visual Display of Quantitative Information*, Cheshire, Graphics Press

Weed L. L. (1969) *Medical Records, Medical Education and Patient Care*, Chicago, Year Book Medical Publishers

Weiss-Lambrou R. (1989) *The Health Professional's Guide to Writing for Publication*, Springfield, Charles C. Thomas

Wells G. (1983) *The Craft of Writing Articles*, London, Allison & Busby

Wells G. (1986) *Writers' Questions Answered*, London, Allison & Busby

Whale J. (1984) *Put it in Writing*, London, J. M. Dent

Young P. (1987) Preliminary steps in writing for publication. *Physiotherapy Practice* 3, 82–84

Bibliography

Allen R. E. (1990) *Oxford Writers' Dictionary*, Oxford, Oxford University Press

Bryson B. (1987) *Dictionary of Troublesome Words*, 2nd edn., Harmondsworth, Penguin

Collinson D. J. *Writing English: a Working Guide to the Skills of Written English*, Aldershot, Wildwood House

Fowler H. W. (1965) *Fowler's Modern English Usage*, 2nd edn., Oxford, Oxford University Press

Kirkpatrick E. M., Schwarz C. M. (1990) *Spell Well!*, Edinburgh, Chambers

Lloyd S. M. (1982) *Roget's Thesaurus*, new edn., London, Longman

Partridge E. (1973) *Usage and Abuse: a Guide to Good English*, Harmondsworth, Penguin

Paxton J. (1986) *Everyman's Dictionary of Abbreviations*, 2nd edn, London, J. M. Dent

Turner B. (1992) *The Writer's Handbook*, London, Macmillan

Wood F. T. (1981) *Current English Usage*, rev. edn., London, Macmillan

Glossary

Abscissa The horizontal (or x) axis on a line chart, frequency polygon or similar two-dimensional figure.

Appendix Subsidiary information attached to the end of a book or document.

Bibliography A list of sources which have been cited and/or are suggested as relevant further reading (see list of references).

Blurb The publisher's description of a book which appears on its cover.

Camera-ready copy Text which has been fully typeset, checked, had tables and figures inserted, and is ready for photographic reproduction by the printer. In some instances, the contract between author and publisher may specify that the author is to provide camera-ready copy.

Cliché A phrase which has become hackneyed through over-use, e.g. to avoid something 'like the plague'.

Continuous scale A scale on which intermediate points or categories can be interpolated between those given on the scale, e.g. age, weight, height (see discrete scale).

Control group   In a controlled trial, the group of subjects which is not exposed to the intervention received by the experimental group (e.g. the control group might receive no treatment, a placebo or a 'standard' alternative to the experimental therapy).

Copy   Textual material intended for printing.

Copy editing   The process whereby the author's manuscript is prepared for the printer. The script is corrected and brought into line with the publisher's house style, and typesetting and similar instructions are inserted for the printer.

Copyright   The exclusive legal right to publish or reproduce a piece of writing or other work.

Correlation   The extent to which two variables vary together. A form of analysis used in inferential statistics.

Defamation   A statement harmful to an individual's reputation which is legally actionable. Such statements are known as libel when written, and as slander when spoken.

Dependent variable   An outcome variable that is measured in the course of a study. The dependent variable is assumed to be influenced by ('depend' upon) another variable, referred to as the independent (or predictor) variable.

Descriptive statistics   The use of statistical techniques to reduce or summarize data (see inferential statistics). Measures of central tendency (e.g. mean) and dispersion (e.g. standard deviation) are examples of descriptive statistics.

Desk-top publishing	The production of high quality written and graphic material, suitable for publication, by means of a computer.
Dichotomous variable	A nominal variable which can take one of two values (e.g. sex).
Discrete scale	A scale on which it is not possible to interpolate intermediate points or categories between those given (e.g. number of children, responses on a Likert scale); also known as a discontinuous scale (see continuous scale).
Dot matrix printer	A printer which forms characters consisting of a patterned series of dots.
Experimental group	In a controlled trial, the group of subjects which is exposed to the experimental condition (see control group).
Figure	Any form of illustration (graph, photograph, line drawing etc.), other than a table.
Floppy disk	A small removable magnetic disk used for storing computer files or software.
Foreword	An introduction to a book written by somebody other than the author(s) (see preface).
Galley proofs	Printed text produced in a strip for checking and correction, prior to being arranged into pages (see page proofs).
Hard copy	Text or graphic material in printed, rather than computerized, form.
Hard disk	A rigid magnetic disk, integral to the structure of a computer, used for storing computer files or software.
Hardware	The equipment that composes a computer system, e.g. disk drive, visual display unit, cables etc.

Harvard reference system A style of bibliographic referencing in which the textual reference is indicated by the author(s) name(s) and the date.

House style A set of conventions adopted by a publisher with respect to layout, spelling, punctuation, referencing etc.

Hypothesis A form of research question stated in the manner of a prediction. The study aims either to retain or reject the hypothesis.

Ibid. An abbreviation for 'ibidem', meaning 'in the same place'; a way of referring to an immediately preceding item in a list of references.

Independent variable See dependent variable.

Inferential statistics The use of statistical techniques to draw conclusions from a set of data. These usually concern inferences made about a population on the basis of data derived from a sample.

Ink-jet printer A printer which forms characters by projecting ink onto the paper through jets.

Interval measurement A level of measurement that gives information as to category, rank and quantity, e.g. IQ, blood pressure readings. Interval measures differ from ordinal in that the distances between adjacent points on the scale are the same in the case of interval measures. The zero point in interval measurement is arbitrary (see nominal, ordinal and ratio measurement).

ISBN International standard book number; a 10-digit number which identifies each book published, usually to be found on the back of the title page.

ISSN

International standard serial number; an 8-digit number which identifies each journal or periodical published.

Justified text

Text which is aligned at the right margin, as well as at the left.

Laser printer

A printer which forms characters by means of a laser beam.

Legend

An explanatory caption for a table or figure.

Libel

See defamation.

Likert scale

A means of measuring attitudes in which a statement is provided to which the respondent indicates one of a number (usually 4 or 5) of standardized, ordinal responses (e.g. strongly agree, agree, no opinion, disagree, strongly disagree).

Linear notes

Notes made in a conventional sequential manner.

List of references

A list of sources to which specific reference has been made in an article, chapter, book etc. (see bibliography).

Loc. cit.

Abbreviation for 'loco citato', meaning 'in the passage cited'; a way of referring to the same page or passage in a previously referenced item in a list of references.

Mean

A form of average arrived at by summing the values of a set of observations and dividing by the number of such observations (see median and mode).

Median

A form of average arrived at by locating the 'middle' value in a rank-ordered series of observations. If there were 13 such observations, the median would be the value of the seventh observation (see mean and mode).

Mode	A form of average arrived at by finding the most frequently-occurring value (see mean and median). A data set may have more than one mode.
Nominal measurement	A level of measurement which only gives information as to category, e.g. male or female, gaseous or liquid (see ordinal, interval and ratio measurement).
Nonparametric statistical tests	See parametric statistical tests.
Op. cit.	Abbreviation for 'opere citato', meaning 'in the work cited'; a way of referring to a previous item in a list of references.
Operational definition	The process whereby a variable is defined in such a way that a) its meaning is specified, b) it is capable of being observed or measured.
Ordinal measurement	A level of measurement which gives information as to category and rank, e.g. working class, middle class, upper class (see nominal, interval and ratio measurement).
Ordinate	The vertical (or y) axis on a line chart, frequency polygon or similar two-dimensional figure.
Outcome variable	See dependent variable.
Page proofs	Printed text arranged into pages, for checking and correction (see galley proofs).
Parametric statistical tests	Tests which require data possessing certain features (e.g. normally distributed and on an interval or ratio scale). Nonparametric tests should be used on data which do not possess these qualities.
Patterned notes	Two-dimensional notes consisting of words or phrases contained within

circles which are linked by radiating lines.

Plagiarism   The act of passing off the literary work of another as one's own, often involving a breach of copyright.

Population   A specified group of people, objects or events from which a sample is drawn. On the basis of the sample, inferences are made as to the population.

Predictor variable   See dependent variable.

Preface   An introduction to a book, written by the author(s) (see foreword). A preface, when present, is generally in addition to, not in place of, an introductory chapter.

Prelims   Introductory pages of a book, including the title page, list of contents, names of contributors etc.

Public lending rights   Payment made to authors whose books are lent in public libraries.

Random sampling   When a sample is taken from a population in such a way that every member of the population has an equal chance of being selected.

Randomization   When subjects are assigned at random to either experimental or control group in a controlled trial; sometimes known as random assignment or random allocation. Each subject has an equal chance of being assigned to either group.

Ratio measurement   A variant of interval measurement in which there is a 'real' zero point, e.g. height, weight (see nominal, ordinal and interval measurement).

Reliability   A research tool is said to possess reliability if it yields consistent measurements on repeated use, by either the same observer or other observers (see validity).

Remaindering   The practice of selling at a reduced price books which have failed to sell at the market rate.

Research question   A statement of the specific area within a topic which a study seeks to explore, e.g. 'how do student therapists perceive the professional status of college tutors in comparison with senior clinical staff?' When a research question takes the form of a prediction, it is referred to as a hypothesis (q.v.).

Roughs   Preliminary sketches produced by an author which are subsequently redrawn by a professional artist.

Royalties   The payment made to authors on the sales of their books, usually as a percentage of the publisher's net receipts.

Sample   See population.

Self-publishing   A method of publishing whereby the author pays for all the costs normally borne by the publisher.

Set-down text   Text which is to appear in a smaller typeface than that used for the major portion of a manuscript.

SI units   Units of measurement specified by the Système International d'Unités (e.g. metre, kilogram, second).

Slander   See defamation.

Standard deviation   A measure of the extent to which scores in a symmetrical (normal) distribution are dispersed around the mean. In such a distribution, 68 per cent of scores lie within one standard deviation either side of the mean; thus the smaller the standard deviation, the more closely scores are grouped around the mean.

Statistical significance A term used when a result is of sufficient magnitude that the possibility of its having come about by chance can be discounted. When the likelihood that a result is due to chance is less than 5 per cent, such a result is generally regarded as being statistically significant (note, however, this is essentially an arbitrary cutoff).

Synopsis A résumé or summary of a proposed book which is sent by an author to a publishing house so that they can assess its suitability.

Table A method of displaying information by means of rows and columns. Entries are made at the intersection of each row and column, in numerical, textual or symbolic form.

Tautology The repetition of a meaning that has already been provided, e.g. 'an unexpected surprise'.

Title page The page of a document which indicates its title and author(s).

Validity A measurement is said to possess validity if it measures what it is supposed to measure and accurate inferences can be drawn from it (see reliability).

Vancouver reference system A style of bibliographic referencing in which the textual references are indicated by consecutive numerals.

Vanity publishing A method of publishing whereby the author makes a contribution to the costs of production.

Word processor A computer whose primary purpose is to compose and edit text.

Index